A HEALING TOUCH

True stories of life, death, and hospice

EDITED BY RICHARD RUSSO

Woodcuts by Siri Beckman

Camden, Maine

ISBN 978-0-89272-751-3

5   4   3   2   1

Printed on acid-free paper by Versa Press, Inc., East Peoria, Illinois

Author royalties, as well as a portion of the proceeds
from sales of this book benefit Hospice Volunteers
of the Waterville Area in Waterville, Maine.

To make a contribution, please contact:
Hospice Volunteers of the Waterville Area
304 Main St.
Waterville, ME 04901
207-873-3615
WWW.HVWA.ORG

Down East

BOOKS·MAGAZINE·ONLINE
www.downeast.com

Distributed to the trade by National Book Network, Inc.

Library of Congress Cataloging-in-Publication Data available on request

CONTENTS

INTRODUCTION

The slender volume you hold in your hand is a collaboration between half a dozen Maine writers and a group of extraordinary people who shared with us their remarkable stories so we could share some of them with you. This book's proceeds go to support the Hospice Volunteers of the Waterville Area (HVWA), and I think readers are going to be surprised—given the shared subject matter (they're all linked to Hospice in some way)—at just how wide-ranging these stories are. They are as varied as the services Hospice provides to its clients, as individual as the people whose experiences are being shared, as stylistically idiosyncratic as the talented writers who recount them. A friend of one of these writers, hearing about our planned project, wondered who'd want to read such a book. For her, as for many people, the word hospice conjures up images of sitting in an overheated, brightly lit room, waiting for someone you love to die. But if you purchased this book, as I hope you have or will, you're going to discover something very different. There's pain and loss, yes, but also laughter and love, faith and hard-won understanding. Life, in other words.

I want to take a moment to name all the people who offered us their stories: Dale Marie Clark, Bill Lord, Leon Duff, Kathy Jenson, Nancy Chamberlain, The Kervin Family (Ed, Sandra, Lori, and Adam), Al and Vicki Hendsbee, Sandy Hussey, Anne Murray Mozingo, Ellen Bowman, Chuck Lakin, Karen Andrews, Ed and Deb Crocker, Donna White, Deb LaVoie, Stan Spoors, Paul LePage, and Tim Robinson. Each took time—in some instances a lot of it—and the telling cost something, often by re-opening old wounds. Sometimes their stories were cathartic, but just as often the tellers found themselves raw and hollowed out after the telling. In the beginning we writers hoped that one in three interviews would yield a story we'd know how to tell. We knew that people were going to open their hearts to us, but we also knew that not every sequence of events, no matter how dramatic, would result in something that feels like a story, something with a beginning, a middle, and an end, something larger than the sum of its parts. But as soon as we started conducting our interviews, we knew we'd underestimated the raw power of such human experience. *Oh my God, how are we ever going to choose which story to write?* we asked each other in panicked phone calls. *They're all so wonderful.* As they were. But we had to choose, and so we did.

How? You might get a slightly different answer depending upon which of us authors you asked, but I think I speak for all of us when I say that the stories we chose to write probably had as much to do with us as the stories themselves. In the end each of us chose the story we thought we understood the best, which may be another way of saying that the experience that was shared with us spoke to us in a way that we felt most competent to relate. When every story moves you deeply, you choose the one you know how to tell best. You'll see what I mean when you move from one story to the next. And I think you'll see something else, too. When I approached my fellow writers with the idea for this project, every one of them said yes in a heartbeat, because the cause was good and because we were being asked to give something we knew how to give. And it was manageable. A few hours worth of interviews, a week or so to write up a draft, another few days to revise. In and out. Except it didn't work out that way. In each of these stories you'll see writers becoming far more involved with their subjects than they imagined would be necessary. The tellers' stories became our own. They intruded into us and we into them. They became too important to get wrong.

And we're glad, since the cause couldn't be better. HVWA serves not just Waterville but twenty-seven nearby towns. Since 1980 its services and programs, all of which are free of charge, have expanded almost exponentially. In 2006 alone the number of clients in the final stages of their lives increased by 70%, participation in grief support groups by 42%, in Camp Ray of Hope by 22%. Hospice volunteers provide companionship visits, respite visits for family, compassionate listening, complementary care sessions, transportation, errand running, reading aloud, and even, as you will learn, music. There are HVWA programs for parents who have lost children, children who have lost parents, for widows and widowers, for women, for men, for whole families. Hospice helps not only the dying but also those who are left behind with the solemn duty to somehow carry on. In other words, all of us. No exceptions. Which means these stories aren't "theirs"; they're ours. All of ours.

Richard Russo
Camden, Maine
December 2007

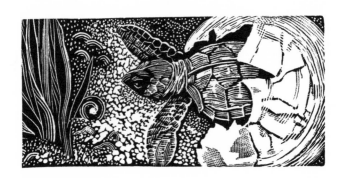

A SON'S GIFT
Gerry Boyle

E d and Debbie Crocker have a good life. One-time high school sweethearts in Old Town, they seem too young to have been married as long as they have—thirty-three years. A former schoolteacher, Ed works in the Sappi paper mill in Skowhegan as a machine tender, monitoring a multimillion-dollar paper machine. He's a friendly, capable guy, the kind who would stop his pickup and help someone broken down beside the road. Debbie went back to school after her children were older and now does the books for Ken's Family Restaurant in Skowhegan. Dark-haired and dark-eyed, she has an engaging directness, a readiness to empathize. She is, as they say, a good listener.

A Healing Touch

Ed has a pilot's license and a small plane, and he and Debbie take flying trips. They've flown as far as Kentucky and Florida. They plan to fly to the midwest in September with Debbie's parents. Their dream trip is to fly their Cessna from Maine to Alaska: Ed hopes that trip is only three or four years away.

The Crockers live in a comfortable contemporary home on Bigelow Hill in Skowhegan. The house is set back from the road in an area of hillside pastures and woods. Before Skowhegan, when their kids were still at home, the couple lived first in Madison and then in Embden, on Embden Pond. Now the kids are grown: Lisa is a hairdresser, 33, married with children. Their son Brandon is 22, married, an engineer on ocean-going tugboats. Aaron, who is 20 and married, too, returned last fall from Iraq where he was crew chief on a U.S. Army Blackhawk helicopter.

And then there is Erik—emphasis on the is. Erik died in a car accident when he was 16. If he were alive today he would be 30. "People ask me, 'How many children do you have?" Debbie said. "It's still four. He's still a part of the family."

The story appeared in the Watervile *Morning Sentinel*, July 26, 1993.

CORNVILLE—A Madison teenager died shortly after midnight Sunday when the car he was driving left Route 43 and slammed into a utility pole.

The victim, Erik Crocker, 16, died instantly from the crash, according to State Trooper Steven Spaulding.

Spaulding said Crocker was headed west about 1-1/2 miles west of Cass Corner when he lost control of the 1987 Chevrolet Nova he was driving.

It crossed the roadway and crashed into the pole on the passenger side, the trooper said, adding there were no passengers.

It took two hours before the Skowhegan Fire Department could remove Crocker, using a power extrication tool, according to Spaulding.

Crews at first had to wait until Central Maine Power crews cut power to the area.

The pole was snapped in half and pulled from the ground by the impact.

Spaulding said a reconstruction of the accident indicates Crocker was driving at least 70 mph in a 45 mph zone.

But speed alone was not a factor.

"There really is no reason why he lost control just because of speed," the state trooper said, noting the area is essentially a straight stretch of roadway.

"There may have been an animal in the road and he tried to avoid it."

There was a strong skunk odor when police arrived to investigate the accident, Spaulding said.

A student at Madison Area Memorial High School, Crocker worked at Ken's Family Restaurant in Skowhegan, was a member of the school tennis team, and was involved in youth ministry at St. Sebastian Roman Catholic Church.

The Crockers make coffee. They pull up chairs in their living room. They start at the beginning, or more precisely, the beginning of the end. Or is it an end that leads to a new beginning?

It was a Saturday. Erik was scheduled to work at the restaurant, 4 p.m. to closing. His mother left in the morning with Brandon and Aaron, then 8, and 10, for a Cub Scout outing at Mt. Blue State Park. "He was home," Debbie said. "He was mowing the lawn. That would be Erik—he would mow until we left and then put the mower away and take off and see his friends before he went to work. Last thing I said to him, 'Make sure you mow that lawn before you go to work.' And that was it."

Ed was working overnight shifts at the mill that

summer. That Saturday, he hadn't seen Erik to talk to in a couple of days. "I remember him telling me he was going somewhere and I never even made eye contact with him," Ed said. "I was sitting there glued to the tube. 'Yup, Erik.'"

The Cub Scout outing was fun. The lawn got mowed. Lisa came by the house and dropped off her daughter Taylor, the Crockers' first grandchild. The baby was two weeks old; it was the first time Lisa had left her with the new grandparents. The younger boys went to bed and around 10 p.m. Lisa came and picked up the baby and went home to Winslow.

Ed and Debbie, with so much to think and talk about as a very good day came to a close, were in bed.

"We'd leave the living room light on for the kids, and they'd have to come upstairs and shut off the light," Debbie said, "and that way we'd know they were home. And we'd go back to sleep. We woke up just a little bit before two and the light was still on. We'd had a talk with him a week or so before about staying out later. We said, 'You're only sixteen.' We woke up and we said, 'That little shit's not home.' So we laid in bed and waited."

It was after 2:00 when they heard a car pull in and stop at the end of the driveway, down by the mailbox,

Ed remembers. "I thought, 'The little shit's gonna try to sneak in. And then—it was a hot summer night, the windows were open—I could hear the radio in the police cruiser. I ran downstairs, I knew that something was wrong. I was still putting my shirt on as I opened up the door. And it was Bob Metivier. Now Bob Metivier was the chief of Troop C [of the Maine State Police]. Well, Bob, I knew him because when I taught at Skowhegan High School, I was also the driver-ed teacher. He used to do accident reconstruction and I would invite him to come to our driver-ed class. So I knew what he did.

"It still hadn't clicked. And he didn't realize [that he knew the family]—we went to the same church, our kids got baptized together—he looked at me and his face dropped. It never clicked. I said, 'Where's Erik?' He said, 'He's at Edwards.' It was Edwards Funeral Home. And then I heard her—she was at the top of the stairs, because she wasn't dressed, she was in her nightgown. I heard her scream like I'd never heard before."

Erik had been accepted at Maine Maritime Academy and planned to join the Merchant Marine. He liked to ski. He loved tennis, played on the school team all three years. He had lots of friends, didn't stick to a high school clique. "Erik's best friend wrote a story about him for graduation night," Debbie says. "One of the things he said was that Erik made friends out of enemies. He was just that kind of kid. No matter where the other child came from or no matter who liked them or didn't like them, he was friends with them."

"Never a problem," Ed says. "Never a problem with him. . . My dad used to tell me I didn't have any patience. I was so quick [to criticize Erik], he was sort of my punching bag. And boy, I'll tell you, when he died, it just killed me."

Debbie adds, "You know, it's your first child and you're young and you want to do everything right."

Ed and Debbie were contacted by someone from Hospice soon after the accident. They were told of the agency's services. Ed and Debbie said they could handle it on their own. They were strong. They would be okay.

"Right," Ed says now.

It turned out that on their own, they were not okay at all.

Debbie recalls that period as just putting one foot in front of the other, a blur, a merry-go-round that went faster and faster. For weeks they barely slept, were so exhausted they were practically passing out on their feet. "You start out maybe two hours a night," Ed says. "A month goes by, you're into three. A couple months go by, you're into four. You are not getting any sleep. Your whole chemistry is different. I could feel my whole nervous system every day."

They got up in the middle of the night, most nights, and had coffee. Read sympathy cards over and over. Debbie couldn't bear to go out even to shop for groceries; she made a list and a friend picked them up. She tried to go back to work but left, unable to answer the question, over and over. "How are you doing?"

People said they were lucky. They still had two boys left. Debbie and Ed didn't feel lucky. They'd lost their son.

That first Thanksgiving they barbecued steak—no turkey. Christmas almost didn't happen. "The first Christmas, she didn't even put a Christmas tree up for the boys," Ed said. "The boys went out and cut this little Charlie Brown tree."

"You could count the needles on the tree—not the branches," Debbie says, smiling.

"They were so proud of it," Ed says. "And they decorated it. There were no lights on it, just construction paper and everything, and a little tinsel. And I'll never forget it. There were two French doors—"

When the holiday was over, the tree was tossed right through them.

"Out that door," Debbie says. "Christmas is over."

For a year, they went to the cemetery every day, sometimes twice, slogging through deep snow that first winter. Ed stopped on the way home from work at five in the morning, knelt at Erik's grave in the dark. "It's pitch black," he says. "I'm on my knees."

Debbie would go to the cemetery and keep vigil on a stone seat they'd brought to the grave site just for that purpose.

"I remember going into the cemetery one day and thinking, I wonder how long it would take me to dig him up. Before anybody noticed. I told Ed. He said, 'What were you going to do with him?' I said, 'I don't know. I just wanted to touch him one more time.' And then, I'm thinking, am I losing it?"

They never went to the scene of the crash, couldn't and wouldn't. But they were drawn to the wrecked car itself, for some reason they had to see it just once. It had been hauled to a local wrecker yard and covered with a tarp.

"We took the tarp off it," Debbie recalls, "and it gave me, I don't know if I can say it was a sense of peace, but I knew that it wasn't gory. There was no blood in the car. Even the gloves of the ambulance attendant were sitting there in the seat. And even though I had seen Erik, it gave me a sense that they were telling me the truth. He was killed instantly. He didn't die hollering for somebody. That was just something I needed to know inside. He didn't need me."

But after his death, she needed him.

Debbie filled her car trunk with Erik's things: sneakers, clothes, his gym bag. She kept them in the car for a full year, would get them out and hold them to her face. It was her refuge, her way to reconnect with the son she had lost. Ed sought a different sanctuary, drinking more and more heavily.

"I lived off Budweiser most of the time. From the time I got up—I was doing shift work—I drank. I was throwing my beer cans behind the back seat of my pickup truck, going to work, then I'd go into the control room, sit there and pass out. Couldn't get along with my co-workers. Didn't care if I got caught. It was amazing how much those people put up with.

"Everything in our marriage—we just didn't get along. What used to work didn't work. We just couldn't get away with it. And then the truth had to come out. We had to get to it, and every time when I started to go to counseling—I almost left her at the counselor's place—I felt like I was being attacked. Of course, drinking came up. I wouldn't want to deal with his death. Just drank, didn't care. You're feeling sorry for yourself, woe is me, and you're just at the bottom.

"And then she didn't feel too well and we weren't getting along too well and I was ready to check out. I didn't give a shit. I kept saying I wanted to get help. We went to HealthReach for a while, the employee assistance program started to work okay for a while, and then you started going back to your old self again. I couldn't deal with her grief, couldn't even handle myself. I certainly couldn't take care of the two kids. The teachers were sending us home their papers. They were writing about their brother they had lost. They were feeling guilty. They used to irritate Erik and get Erik mad and then get in a fight and we were always picking on Erik, 'Leave them alone. Leave the two little ones alone.'"

And then Ed did hit bottom—almost.

He was sitting on his bed one day, he remembers, and he was thinking about the hunting rifle just a few feet away. It seemed to be the only way out of his grief, the excruciating depths of his sadness. "My .308 was in my closet, and I got so close," he says. "Couldn't see anything. You can't. A person who is going to take his life, I really believe he cannot see what devastation he's going to create for the others. The world closes in so much. You get so tunnel-visioned, you can't see that. All you know is that you're in so much pain and you can't take any more and you just want to end it. That's all you can see."

Sometimes, though, a glimmer of light filters through the suffocating darkness.

For the Crockers, ironically, the catalyst was another tragedy, this one monumental and wrenchingly close to home.

It was September 14, 1994, a year and two months after Erik's death. Five teenagers from the town of Athens were on their way to school in neighboring Madison—Erik's school. They drove out of town that morning and headed west on Route 43, past occasional houses, a big dairy farm, passing the place—the utility pole now replaced—where Erik died. Two miles down the road, at the intersection of Route 43 and Route 201, known locally as Twelve Corners, the driver pulled into the path of a northbound dump truck. The truck driver couldn't stop; the car was struck broadside and thrown fifty feet. Three of the teenagers were dead at the scene. The other two died later that day.

"And they were all friends of Erik's," Debbie Crocker said. "I picked up the phone after that and I said, 'Okay, I guess I can't do this alone.' When something like that happens it puts you right back to where you were really quick." The overwhelming grief. The paralyzing sense of loss.

Debbie called Hospice, and was told there was a group for parents who had lost children. She went for a year—alone. "He was still pretty stubborn and was not going to sit with a bunch of women and talk about our son," she said.

And then she was told about a new program called Camp Ray of Hope, about to be launched by Hospice Volunteers of Waterville. It was going to take place over a weekend in September at a camp in Winthrop. No way was Ed going. But as the date approached, and Debbie announced she was going to go and take Brandon and Aaron, too, Ed grudgingly relented. Turned out he was the only man there; he wanted to bail out, go stay in a motel.

But he stayed. He did talk about his son, but first he sat and listened as two women in the group spoke. They had lost their husbands.

"One of them," he says, "I'm sitting in that group and she starts to tell her story, and her husband has committed suicide at their favorite lookout. She was suspicious something was wrong. He hadn't been talking the last couple of weeks. She got a call from work; he hadn't shown up. She decided to see if he was up there—and he'd blown his brains out.

"And she had two little children. And I can just remember the crying, her telling her story, and I'm trying to hold it in, and you just knew this was so real, it was no setup. And then the next lady starts talking—and guess what? Those kids watched [their father] die. He drank himself to death. And he was the nicest man and the nicest father, but he had a drinking problem."

At that moment Ed stopped drinking, he says. He stopped feeling sorry for himself. "I was woken up in a one-hour session," Ed says. "I never forgot it."

Debbie adds, "It was kind of like God put you in a place."

The Crockers went back to Camp Ray of Hope the next year. They've attended most years since, first as participants and then as facilitators. They have seen the camp grow from three couples to more than sixty.

Debbie has been trained to facilitate groups for grieving parents and Ed is planning to take the training,
too. "A lot of parents," she says, "they say, 'If you can
look at another parent and think, okay, they're still
here. They're sane. We can do this. It's going to take a
lot of hard work."

For Debbie and Ed it has taken just that.

"It was still a slow process because now we had to
rebuild our relationship," Ed says. "For the first time
we tore the wall down and it didn't come back up.
Now we had to start it all over and trust each other, to
believe in each other. There was no more garbage stuff.
All the old stuff that we used to fight about—off
limits. We'd either get through it and accept it for what
it is or learn to listen.

"I don't like to fight. I don't like to argue anymore.
I had to learn to count to ten. I always felt I had to
have an answer."

Debbie smiles. "He just wanted to fix everything.
He just wanted to fix all of the grief and just wanted it
to go way. He couldn't fix it. He couldn't fix it for the
kids. He couldn't fix it for himself. You can't fix it.
There's no method."

"I'm fortunate that I've made it to this point," her
husband says. "Some people never would. They would

be like this for the rest of their lives. Everybody says, well it's time to move on. You never know. If it takes eight years to stop grieving, it takes eight. If it takes ten, it takes ten. Whatever it takes. Everybody is different."

And in an indication of their closeness, they speak in alternating sequence, back and forth, like singers taking solos.

Debbie: "I can go on and be there for other people and share what I've felt, what's worked and what doesn't work for me. But there's no fix. I'll always miss him."

Ed: "Me, too. That's one thing, we can still hear his voice. That's the one thing. It's him coming in the door, with them big feet, saying, 'I'm hungry, what's to eat?' I can still hear that sound."

Debbie: "We lived in a raised ranch. He'd come up the stairs and he'd take them about three at a time because he was tall. 'Hey guys, what's to eat?' Head right for the kitchen, that was his first stop. He'd open his eyes in the morning and he'd head right for the kitchen."

It's a treasured memory, but others, seen with new clarity, are more difficult to relive. For Ed it is the acknowledgment that he was tough on his eldest son.

"I was so hard on him," he says, with a rueful smile. "We're out there hunting, walking in the leaves, and I'll betcha I'm making just as much noise as that poor kid. And he's looking at me. Poor kid's trying to learn. I look back at him—that one hurts me so bad. I can laugh at it now, thankfully."

He pauses.

"Oh, he was such a punching bag. And he'd always try to please me."

And now, in a way, the roles are reversed.

"People say, 'Oh, you're fortunate because you have two more kids [to raise],'" Ed says. "That's a hard one, because nobody can replace Erik. But now I can look at it and say they have been my lifesaver. To help me go on, but also, what a lucky man I am to have a second chance to be a better father."

He has tried to be just that. When Erik was young, Ed would be off snowmobiling. Erik wanted to play softball or baseball and Ed was too busy. He changed that with his younger sons. Instead of snowmobiling, Ed and Debbie attended the younger boys' ski races, standing for hours on the side of the trail, waiting for a glimpse of one of their sons flashing through the gates.

He tries to be patient. To listen. Fourteen years

after his death, Erik is not gone. He is there, showing Ed how to be a better father, a better person.

Some people advise parents to dispose of all of their child's things, but Debbie counsels grieving parents to do whatever feels right. She still keeps the box of Erik's belongings in the basement. "His socks, his underwear, his aftershave. Nobody touches that. If I want to smell him, I open it up and smell it. I'm all set."

Ed, who once visited the cemetery twice a day, who knelt at his son's grave in the dark, now visits once or twice a year. He doesn't have to go to the gravesite because his son is with him. "He is my rock today," Ed said. "I try to build my strength through him, to try to be a better father, a better husband. I can't believe I've come as far as I have. I attribute it to Camp Ray of Hope. It's not the miracle for everybody. I was just fortunate."

Miracle, yes. Panacea, no.

They talk about him often. They visit the grave—with its black-granite stone engraved with a deer, birch trees, Erik's tennis racquet—once or twice a year. On his birthday—August 31—Debbie makes a pumpkin pie—Erik didn't like cake—and she puts a candle in it. They no longer sing.

"I'll shed tears," Debbie says. "Sometimes I'll hear a song and it will be like it was that day again. But the peaks and valleys aren't as deep. The valleys aren't as deep and you can come out of them quicker. And I do have a lot of good days. I have a lot of laughter when I think of things that he did. I miss him greatly. Weddings. Babies. I look at his picture. The last picture I had of him, he was sixteen years old. What would he look like now? Where would he be? What would he be doing? Those are things that still come and eat at your insides.

She pauses.

"But I can honestly say that I am extremely thankful that I was given the gift of him for sixteen years. And even if I knew that I was going to lose him, I wouldn't have hesitated for a moment to have him."

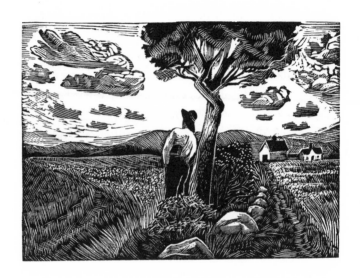

YOU KNOW
WHO YOU ARE

Richard Russo

I met Lee Duff over a decade ago at a place called Champions when I was teaching at Colby College in Waterville. There were no champions at Champions, at least none I recall, but there were some pretty fair racquetball players. Lee was one, I another. Lee's game was a lot like Lee: pragmatic, resourceful, buoyantly optimistic. Beat him fifteen to two in the first game of the match and he'll take the ball, stride to the service line, point his racket at you and say, "Your ass is mine." Then, having served notice, he serves the ball, and if you're not ready, too damn bad. The last thing he wants is for you to savor your victory. There's work to be done and he's just the man to do it. When he gets the lead, he announces the score as if through a bullhorn, an unsubtle reminder of whose property your ass is (not yours). To his way of thinking, the fact that I'm fifteen years his junior is a minor inconvenience. He's beaten me before, so why not again? His joy in what transpires on that court, win or lose, is bounded only by its walls. "Trombones!" he bellows, when he goes ahead seven to six. I'd been playing with him a good month before I caught on to that particular allusion (*76 Trombones*, get it? get it?).

It was clear from the start that we both derived the same benefit from sport in general, and racquetball in particular. "It drains the poison," was the way Lee liked to put it, and I knew just what he meant. As a writer and teacher, I spent most of my time living in my head and trying to get my students to live in theirs, or to at least visit those heads now and then. Lee spent much of his time suffering fools, something he didn't do gladly but was part of his unofficial job description as superintendent of schools in nearby China/Vassalboro/Winslow. In the winter (half the school year in central Maine) when snow was a possibility (often), his day began at four in the morning, by which time he had to be up listening to the weather service reports in order to decide whether circumstances warranted canceling school. Canceling and not canceling it got him pretty much the same reward, a torrent of abuse from parents, teachers, and bus drivers. When school got out, there'd be a different set of challenges: budget meetings, policy meetings, parent group meetings, individual parent meetings, school board meetings, disciplinary meetings (of both the student and teacher variety). As an academic, I knew all about meetings, and knew that Lee had it far worse than I did.

In the middle of the day, though, three days a week, there was the oasis of racquetball, a quick, furious, very physical sport that demands concentration and anticipation. If you don't anticipate your opponent's forehand, for instance, and step in front of his shot, the ball will raise a welt the size of a small orange on your tender backside. It hurts like hell, but it's pleasurable indeed compared to an irate parent explaining why you're a moron for canceling school on a day when it didn't snow as much as predicted. Sympathy—Lee likes to remind me, is located in the dictionary between *shit* and *syphilis*.

Lee grew up on a dairy and potato farm near Houlton, Maine, the ninth of ten siblings, facts that go a long way toward explaining his pragmatism, if not his optimism. I don't know where the latter comes from, and I doubt Lee does either. New England is not known for begetting optimists, and northern Maine's shallow, hardscrabble soil and long, bitter winters are more likely to make you a Calvinist or a Red Sox fan or, tragically, both. When Lee was seven, he already had adult responsibilities on the farm. Three of his older brothers and one sister were serving overseas in the Second World War, which meant that much of their work fell to him. Even at that young age, he worked six days a week. Up at the crack of dawn or before, he had to milk the cows before school started, and after school there were endless homework-preventing chores. He attended a one-room school that housed kindergarten through eighth grade, and like most farm kids, he lost two or three weeks every autumn to the harvest and another two or three in the spring to planting. All of which explains why Lee, despite having a genuinely curious mind and lively intellect, was a mediocre student. He tells a story that goes a long way toward explaining the kind of man he would later become.

When he was ten, one of his many jobs was driving the tractor, and one particular autumn found him harrowing a field long after dark. It was bitter cold, frightening work for a kid, all alone on a tractor, traveling over unlevel terrain. The tractor's headlamp shone off into black woods that surrounded the sloping field on three sides, occasionally locating bright eyes among the trees. A cat's eyes? A dog's? A deer's? A bear's? No, probably not a bear's, but maybe. If it was a bear, could he outrun it? No. Even trying would risk death or dismemberment. You don't jump down from a tractor in the dark, not when it's trailing a harrow. Lee doesn't remember how much of the field he'd worked when the pin that attached the harrow to the tractor either broke or popped free, but he heard it go and felt the harrow detach. He also knew that it was pointless to search in pitch darkness for a pin that was probably broken anyway. He knew his father would not be pleased, but what choice did he have? There was nothing to do but drive the tractor home. He remembers thinking, "I can't reverse what's happened. I can't control it. It's gone."

When he got home, his father was more than displeased. You don't come home with the job undone, he explained. Life demanded that you be resourceful. Problems had solutions. He should have found a way. He'd not only failed, he'd done the one unforgivable thing: he hadn't tried. Another kid would have resented the unfairness of such criticism. First, was it even true that every problem had a solution? More to the point, wasn't the solution to the present problem more likely to reveal itself in the morning, in the light of day? Lee might have raised these points but did not. He understood his father knew perfectly well he was being unfair, but was also trying to teach him something about life, which could be far more unjust than an angry but caring parent. Problems might seem insurmountable, but in the end they were just problems. When you don't know what to do, you try something. If that doesn't work, you try something else. You keep trying. You don't come home until the job is done.

When Lee told me this story, I couldn't help thinking how different my own life experiences had been as a kid. I'd not been overburdened with adult responsibilities, or any responsibilities, really, except for doing well in school, but somehow I'd arrived at many of the same conclusions about the best way of dealing with life's problems and inequities. "Do *some* goddamn thing, even if it's wrong," my own father always used to say, usually right before doing the wrong thing, but in this respect I was very much his son. I hated both inaction and the caution that led to it. And I had a formative story of my own.

When I was a freshman in high school, my friends and I often stopped at this one particular market on the way home from school. There was a clerk there who liked to give us a hard time, a pseudo-intellectual fellow who was forever insinuating we were none too bright. One day, to demonstrate this thesis, he gave us a puzzle to solve. It was a kind of pyramid, wide at the bottom and narrow at the top, made up of rectangular boxes. He drew it for us on a piece of paper. You could start anywhere you wanted, inside or outside the pyramid. Your task was to draw a continuous line through each side of every box, but having crossed a line you weren't allowed to cross it a second time. My friends and I worked on the puzzle for the rest of the afternoon without success. "It can't be done," one of my friends assured me, by which I understood him to mean that it was difficult. A month later I was still trying to solve the pyramid, and probably wouldn't have given up even then if the smirking store clerk hadn't finally taken pity and let me in on the secret: *there was no solution to the puzzle*. He'd set us an impossible task for the pure pleasure of watching us fail.

But here's something to consider: The truth doesn't always set you free. I wasn't sure I believed him. Did he know there was no solution, as he claimed? Or had he just not found it? I was pretty sure I was smarter than he was and kept imagining the look on his face when I showed him how I'd succeeded in doing what he claimed was impossible. Hubris, sure, but it went beyond that. The puzzle had become part of the ritual of my days. Giving it up meant not just defeat but loss. If I no longer had the puzzle, what was there to replace it? Even now, as an adult, I still remember that pyramid with something like affection. It may even have been part of my early training to write novels, an activity that places a premium on both patience and dogged resourcefulness in the face of seeming impossibility. You don't know what to do far more often than you do, which is why the novelist's mantra is, or should be: *Try something. If it doesn't work, try something else. Keep trying. There is a solution.* What if there isn't? That's a question every good novelist knows better than to ask.

By the time Lee and I met, life had taught us that there *were* problems without solutions. But it had also taught us that complex problems with difficult solutions often look for all the world like impossible problems with no solutions. The trick is to know the difference, and often the only way to be sure is to try. Compared to giving up, it's a healthy and productive philosophy that's likely to build character. It works. Until one day it doesn't. Then you're in for a bad time, because your greatest strength becomes a weakness, your primary character asset a liability. Your reluctance to give up, to admit defeat, to recognize futility for what it is now guarantees that you will suffer more than you need to.

One day in 1994 Lee came home from school and was surprised to discover that Ann, his wife, was not there. Had he forgotten a meeting? They both had very busy schedules. She was a tireless volunteer at their church, and her fair-mindedness and industry made her much sought-after when it came to committees. Lee himself had just gotten out of one meeting and he'd come home for a quick bite to eat before driving back in to town for another. It was odd, though. Usually, Ann left a note if they weren't going to eat dinner together, and there wasn't one. Nor was there a message from her on the answering machine, and the house didn't feel like she'd been there recently. He was talking himself out of becoming anxious when he heard her pull in. A couple of minutes later, when Ann came into the kitchen, she looked more puzzled than worried. "Funny thing just happened," she told him. "I couldn't remember how to get home."

Ann Barnes grew up in Houlton, Maine, the middle of three children, about five miles from the Duff potato/dairy farm, either that or a world away, depending on how you measure these things. Hers was a distinguished Maine family. Her grandfather, who studied privately with Oliver Wendell Holmes, had been chief justice of the Maine Supreme Court, despite never having attended law school. Her father was a county attorney who became a Maine Senator and Speaker of the House. That's aristocracy in northern Maine, or anywhere in Maine, probably anywhere in New England. The Barneses were liberal Baptists who placed a premium on education, providing in both respects a contrast to the Duffs, who belonged to what Lee remembers with a wry smile as a "strict country church," as unyielding and unforgiving in its orthodoxy as the shallow, rocky soil they tilled. Of course one of the beauties of living in a place as sparsely populated as northern Maine, at least if you like the idea of democ-

racy and all that it implies, is that rich or poor, edu-
cated or uneducated, aristocratic or plebian, there's a
good chance you'll end up in the same school. Once
there, you might meet somebody different from yourself. She might be beautiful. You might fall in love with
her. You might stay in love with her for the rest of your
life. Because as good as class and religion and education and money are at establishing boundaries, human
nature is even better at defying them.

The Ricker Classical Institute in Houlton was such
a place. One hundred kids. Four grades. Lee and Ann
met there and dated throughout high school. Ann's father was impressed with young Lee Duff's sobriety and
industry, his seriousness, and, yes, his resourcefulness.
"Is there anything you *can't* do?" Ann's father once
asked him, amazed by Lee's versatility. But then the
man hadn't grown up on a farm, where plumbing, elec-
trical, woodworking, and engine repair are all part of
everyday life. So, sure, he was impressed.

He also liked the fact that Lee not only loved his
daughter, but also respected her. He knew his daughter could do worse. Still, in his heart of hearts, did he
also believe she could do better? There was, after all,
the whole wide world, and what father wouldn't want
his daughter to see some of it before settling on a local

boy? If Ann confided to her father that she loved young Lee Duff, that she thought maybe he might be the one, that she was never truly happy except when they were together, could he be blamed for letting her in on a little secret—that this was the way love *always* felt, that it could feel that way more than once?

Who could blame him if he looked forward to high school being over? Then his daughter would be heading off to Colby College, his *alma mater,* a prestigious and expensive liberal arts college in Waterville, Maine, and Lee to evangelical Bob Jones University in South Carolina where his siblings had gone. Then both time and distance, which also had been known to construct durable barriers against human nature, would be on his side.

But of course I'm guessing. Maybe to Ann's father, Lee's decency, industry and generosity were full and sufficient recommendation. Maybe he wanted only his daughter's happiness and was untroubled by things like class and money and religious upbringing, things that have bedeviled other fathers down through the ages. Every father wants his daughter to be happy; not very many have the ability to separate their own notions of happiness from hers. At any rate Lee sometimes suspected that Ann's parents thought she was "dating down," but he liked her family and was grateful that they seemed to like him, too. That he and Ann should go their separate ways for a while after high school seemed reasonable.

One more thing to know about the Barnes family: They had a history of Alzheimer's.

He knew. Right from the start, some part of Lee knew. Ann's forgetting how to get home was not "a funny thing," and now he began to recall other incidents. Of late, Ann had seemed uncharacteristically absent-minded. She'd walk off and leave a stove burner on in the kitchen. Opening a kitchen cabinet, Lee would discover something that belonged in the pantry, and when he went to put it there he'd find something else that belonged in the kitchen cabinet. Such mishaps were minor, insignificant in and of themselves, but now he had to consider another terrible possibility. Had Ann simply forgotten to turn off the burner, or did she not remember its ever having been on? Was she hurriedly putting things in the wrong place, or could she not remember where they went?

There was a difference, and Lee knew, deep down, what the difference was, that it had a name. But it wasn't a name that could be spoken out loud, at least not yet. And there was another thing he was sure of. Ann knew too. Only fifteen years earlier she'd gotten a call from her older brother, asking her and Lee to drive to Houlton to help assess her father's condition, which at the time was often called "hardening of the arteries." But it was Alzheimer's, an aggressive case, and by the time the family convened, her mother was black and blue from trying to deal with him. Ann and Lee had been instrumental in convincing her mother there was no way she could handle her husband any longer.

A month after the first, there was a second driving incident. This time he and Ann were returning home from Houlton in separate cars, Lee leading, Ann following. Lee noticed she kept falling behind. Even in his rearview mirror, Ann's driving didn't seem right. Worried, he pulled over onto the shoulder and she, blessedly, did too. Getting out, he found her, pale and rigid with terror, gripping the steering wheel as if her life depended on it, even with the car at rest. She'd forgotten not just how to drive, but how the car worked, what made it go faster, what slowed it, what turned it off. The harder she thought, the more foreign everything in the car seemed. It was all too complicated, as if, in the blink of an eye, a child's game of Chutes and Ladders had become a Rubik's Cube.

Frightened out of his own wits, Lee nevertheless knew that the first thing to do was diminish, if possible, Ann's panic, no easy task when his own was rising. But he took her hand and went into a catcher's crouch there on the shoulder of the road, telling her to relax, that they weren't in any hurry to get home. If she was too frightened to drive, he could come back for the car later. "I'm worried," she confessed. "I don't know what's happening."

"I'm worried, too," he admitted, but he assured her that everything would be all right. Probably she'd just suffered a panic attack. How long did they remain there along the side of the road, holding hands? Lee doesn't remember. But after a while the knowledge of how to drive a car was there again, so simple, the gas pedal to make the car go, the brake to slow and stop it, the key in the ignition to start it up. So simple.

Lee and Ann were married in Houlton, Maine, in 1957. Ann had gone off to Colby as planned but after a couple years transferred to the University of Connecticut, where she could study nursing, a program that Colby didn't offer. She was a good, industrious student, just as she'd been in high school, and she joined singing groups and acted in plays. Also as planned, Lee went to Bob Jones, where he was also a good and popular student. Neither dated. They wrote each other long letters in which they looked forward to the Christmas holiday or summer vacation, when they would be together again. Not just together. Inseparable. And so no one was surprised when, during their senior year, despite the obstacles of time and distance, despite those differences in religion, education, and class, they became engaged. People who love each other can be damned stubborn.

Well, there was one problem, at least for Ann, and it came to a head when she went to South Carolina for Lee's graduation. Ann was, had always been, an introvert. She was no shrinking violet, but was by nature both quiet and shy, and while she possessed excellent social skills, she never put herself forward, never sought the limelight, never was the first to laugh. Of course she knew that the man she was engaged to was the farthest thing from an introvert. He was not just the first person to laugh but also the second. Put Lee in a roomful of strangers and he'd find a conversation before he'd hung up his coat. He'd leave knowing everyone. In Houlton, Maine, Lee's outgoing ways hadn't been a problem because they knew the same people and were comfortable with most of them. Over time Ann had made small circles of close friends at UConn, but at Bob Jones she discovered that Lee knew everyone and everyone knew him. People sought him out, consulted him, seemed to need him in order to accomplish much of anything. Worse, he wanted to introduce her to every single one of them. And, naturally, they were curious about what sort of girl had captivated him so completely. They imagined she must be a female version of himself, another force of nature, who'd match him joke for joke, idea for idea, plan for plan. For the entire graduation weekend the spotlight she'd always shunned fell blindingly on her, a deer in the headlights.

On the drive back to Maine, she gave Lee his ring back, explaining that she didn't think they really knew each other very well, by which he understood her to mean that she didn't know him very well, and maybe there was even more to it than that. It seemed to him that Ann was more troubled by what she did know about her fiancé than what she didn't. What she'd just been offered at Jones was a glimpse of what life might be like if she married an extrovert like Lee Duff. Hell was what it might be like. A life of endless introductions and frightening social expectations for which she was ill-equipped. But she was no sooner back in New Haven and more familiar surroundings than Ann realized she'd made a mistake, because there Lee was just Lee again: kind, full of fun, utterly devoted. She'd allowed herself to be spooked by the novelty and heightened drama of the experience. No doubt the future would hold many more new experiences, but the question was, in whose company did she wish to face that future? She knew the answer. She'd known it for a long time. By mid-summer the engagement was back on.

That fall Ann would enter the final year of her five-year nursing program, much of it at Yale/New Haven Hospital, but Lee was now armed with a brand-new teaching degree. If he could land a job, they could get married. As it happened there were three area positions advertised for junior high school social studies/ English teachers in the New Haven area, and Lee applied for all three. The best was in New Haven itself and in short order the life skill that had so frightened Ann in South Carolina—Lee's ability to make friends of strangers— paid its first dividend. At the end of the interview he was offered the job. He called her at her dormitory with the news and drove over to pick her up. They went directly to a beach in East Haven, where, as they walked back and forth in the sand, they set a date and planned the wedding and the rest of their lives. The sun was still high when they'd started, long set by the time they finished their talking and planning and Lee reluctantly took Ann back to the dorm. She was late and would catch hell, but she didn't care.

With most life-threatening illnesses early diagnosis is key and being young is advantageous. Not so Alzheimer's. The younger a person is when diagnosed, the more precipitous the physical and mental decline is likely to be, and catching the disease early gets you nothing. Ann's reluctance to talk about what was happening to her prevented any official diagnosis until spring of that first year when her symptoms became undeniable. It was their grown daughter Kathy, who lived in the area, that finally convinced Lee to take her in to be evaluated, and it was then that the word they'd been unwilling to speak was finally said out loud. Ann was diagnosed with early advent Alzheimer's, and the diagnosis had an immediate and profound effect. She began a gradual withdrawal from everyday life, as if the word she'd dreaded for months now gave her permission to be ill, to acknowledge what until now she'd felt obliged to deny. Her decline now began in earnest.

For Lee the hardest part of that decline was the almost immediate loss of verbal intimacy. Within two short years Ann would go from confusing similar-sounding words to not communicating at all. Their marriage, like so many strong marriages, had been centered in language. They'd always made a ritual of the evening meal, during which their talk was as nourishing as the food they ate; talk was how they made sense of their time apart. Nothing that happened to them during the day was ever completely real until it was recounted, shared, evaluated. The day's delights, its outrages, its hilarity, its challenges, its significance—all of it was fodder for evening conversation, for the necessary planning of tomorrow. Strategy. Reassurance. Laughter. The language of devotion, of commitment.

Though it was difficult, Lee could bear the fact that Ann could no longer drive or cook or play bridge or contribute much to running the house, but it was beyond dispiriting to realize that he could no longer tell her about his day—the school board meeting that had, despite his best efforts, devolved into an angry shouting match, or the teacher and friend he was going to have to fire, or the secretary at the middle school who had once again arrived at work with a black eye and busted lip, courtesy of her husband. Such revelations now produced in Ann a disproportionate response, often abject terror. So did smaller annoyances: misplaced objects, a window that wouldn't shut right. Lee had to be careful never to raise his voice, never to allow his concerns, his fears, no matter how real, to register on his face, lest they occasion great distress. Once his confidant in all things, Ann now needed to be told, repeatedly, in word and gesture, that everything was fine, that there was nothing to fear. And so it was that a relationship based on shared truth and trust suddenly became one that relied on well-intentioned, benign lies. Lee's own growing distress, his plummeting spirits, had to remain hidden at all costs.

Even worse than Ann's failures of memory were her brief periods of terrible lucidity. As her condition worsened, she became more confused, frightened, and angry than she'd ever been. Her sudden inability to do things she'd been doing since she was a child was not lost on her, at least not all of the time. One morning when she was trying to dress herself, Lee saw that she was becoming more and more frustrated, but when he tried to help her, she turned on him in a fury, "Why don't you just shoot me?" An hour later, of course, she didn't remember having said those words, had no memory of the frustration that had occasioned them. But they were words Lee would never forget. That's one of the disease's many cruel ironies—that one person's inability to remember will cause things to happen that are forever etched in the brain of that person's caregiver. No blessed forgetting for him. Not ever.

In the beginning money was tight. Thanks to its proximity to New York City and that vast economic weather pattern known as Yale University, New Haven wasn't a cheap place to live. They rented a third-floor flat in a racially mixed neighborhood where burglaries were common but which otherwise was relatively safe. They never went out to eat and Lee vividly remembers that one month the balance in their checking account was $3.21. He bought a used 1951 Ford sedan and discovered that by shoveling just enough to get out when it snowed he could, in effect, save the parking space in front of their apartment.

It was a time of discovery. Among other things, he and Ann were discovering and inventing their marriage, the way every newlywed couple must, figuring out who would be responsible for what. Ann, who had far less experience pinching pennies than her husband, nevertheless took over the books and in no time proved she was the right person for the job. She always knew where every cent was, where the next was coming from, whether there would be enough of them to cover both foreseeable and unpredictable expenses. She also proved expert at finding good, inexpensive, nutritious food. She would have need of such rigorous managerial skills, because their first son, Bruce, was born a year after they wed, making things really interesting. In short order another child followed, and Ann quit her part-time nursing job.

Lee taught junior high for three years in New Haven, then another three in nearby North Haven, during which time he enjoyed the classroom, though he was beginning to suspect that his real calling was administration. That would pay more, for one thing, but money wasn't really the issue. Ever the pragmatist, nothing appalled Lee more than a poorly run program. Thanks to those early years on the family farm, the urge to fix anything that was broken came as naturally to Lee Duff as breathing. Unfortunately, you don't get promoted into administration by virtue of being a good teacher or even by demonstrating an aptitude for making things run smoothly. For that, as in *The Wizard of Oz,* you need a diploma, or, in

Lee's case, certification. To qualify for an assistant principal post, he'd have to go back to graduate school; at the time the three-credit certification course at UConn cost ninety dollars, money he knew they didn't have.

But to his surprise, when he broached the subject of continuing his education with Ann, she didn't hesitate. By then she knew her husband, knew what he was good at, just as she knew how people gravitated to him, trusted him, were willing to work with and for him. None of that frightened her anymore. They would find the money. And then Lee caught a break, one that not everybody in his position would have recognized as good fortune. His first job as an assistant principal was under the supervision of a principal who was on his way out the door, just a few short years from the official retirement he'd already unofficially embarked upon. Which meant that Lee was free to do what he'd been wanting to do for years. Take a few risks. Break a few rules. Try something. If that didn't work, try something else. There was no shortage of problems in junior high schools. He had to believe that most of them had solutions. He was on the case.

Memory. Most adults suffer some loss as they get older. My grandmother was sharp as a tack well into her eighties, but when she got excited she'd forget the names of her loved ones, especially mis-behaving grandchildren. Anxious to reprimand us, she first had to get the attention of whoever had transgressed. *Rick, Greg, Cathie, Johnny, Carole, Jimmy*. Down she'd scroll through our names, some-times mixing in the names of her daughters, her husband, other relatives and friends. All the while the guilty kid would be standing there grinning at her, confident that there could be no punishment until the perp's identity was fixed, though some-times, if the right name could not be located, my grandmother would point her arthritic index finger at you and say, "You know who you are!" Such small tricks of the mind are often like that, comic to all but the person whose mind is playing the trick.

When the tricks the mind plays are larger, the re-sults can be terrifying. Some years ago my mother, then in her late seventies suffered an episode of temporary dementia brought on by some warring medications, the problem exacerbated by the fact that we were just then moving from Waterville to the Maine coast and she was in unfamiliar surroundings. We made an appointment with a doctor, but when I arrived at her apartment, she was still in her robe, and I could see immediately that she was in a state of panic. "What time is it?" she wanted to know, which led me to believe the exhaustion resulting from the move had caused her to oversleep and now she'd be late for her first visit with a new doctor. But when I told her the time, she bolted across the room at unsafe speed for a woman of her years and wrote what I told her onto a piece of paper, under which she printed in bold letters and underlined: REAL TIME. Then she sat down, visibly relieved. When I asked why she'd written down the time, her chilling reply was that later in the day she'd want to know what time it was, and now she'd have that information at her fingertips. When I looked around her new living room, I saw that every clock in it registered a different time.

For the Alzheimer's patient the world is full of such impenetrable confusions, and they don't get resolved the way my mother's confusion about the nature of time did when her new doctor got her medications straightened out. For the Alzheimer's sufferer the world becomes foreign, incomprehensible, as the familiar morphs by degrees into the unfamiliar, the strange, the incomprehensible. For that person's caregiver, the world may not be foreign, but it's equally nightmarish. Caregivers, in addition to keeping the world safe for the sufferer, also serve as interpreters of a world gone haywire. I had just a glimpse of that (all I wanted, believe me) as I sat in the doctor's office with my mother that morning, trying, without success, to help her understand why the minute hand on her watch traveled in one direction (clockwise, a term that's of little use as explanation) and never the reverse. She didn't understand why, if this was her watch, she couldn't make time operate according to her wishes. Finally, she succeeded in breaking the stem, which satisfied her as completely as writing down the time on a slip of paper had done earlier.

But here's the even more surprising thing: what I remember thinking was that although the woman sitting next to me was undeniably my mother, she was also somehow not my mother for the simple reason that my mother knew how time worked and this woman did not. In other words, what she'd forgotten during the night had stolen some measure of her identity, and it wasn't until two days later, when her memory of how time worked returned, that she was wholly my mother again.

And so it was for Lee during much of that first year after Ann was diagnosed. There she was, right before his eyes, his wife, his lover, his friend, the mother of his children, and yet she was also departing, day after day, one memory at a time, like a photograph left out in the sun, fading into whiteness. As Ann's withdrawal from the details of everyday life deepened, he began to understand the link between memory and identity, that we are all, in a sense, not so much the sum of our experiences as the sum of our memories of them. Some things we can forget without great consequence because they are not us. Ann had always loved to play bridge, but when she lost that ability she didn't cease to be Ann. But all too soon she was forgetting other things.

Where elderly people with dementia suffer a gradual decline, Ann was not elderly and her decline, as predicted, was both steep and terrifying. Within months she was beginning to forget the kinds of things you wouldn't think a human being *could* forget: what knives and forks are for, how to brush your teeth, the difference between food, which can be eaten, and the plate it rests upon, which cannot, how to swallow the food you've chewed, who the man is who's feeding you, who you, the person doing the chewing, are. (*You know who you are!* my grandmother had insisted.) And Ann's was not the only identity under attack. "Who am I," Lee often wondered, "if I'm not this woman's husband?"

It was during the second year of Ann's precipitous decline that I witnessed a snapshot of his private, on-going hell. I knew he was struggling. Who wouldn't be? He'd lost twenty pounds, and he'd become visibly stooped under the weight he was carrying. But we'd continued our two or three times a week racquetball matches, during which he tried as best he could to drain at least some of the poison. I generally didn't ask about Ann unless he volunteered. I knew that our racquetball matches were an escape, that it would be no kindness to return him to the reality he was fleeing, however temporarily. But this particular day he was clearly not himself, his usual buoyancy flown. In the first game the score had been seven to six, but there'd been no trombones. So, halfway through the match, while we rested outside the court, I inquired.

That morning, he confided, before he left for work, he'd noticed that Ann's face didn't look right, something about her cheeks. The woman who looked after her while Lee was at work, who would make breakfast as soon as she arrived, was running a few minutes late. In fact, he heard the woman's car pulling up in the drive as he went over to where Ann stood and asked her to open her mouth, which she did. "She stood there with her mouth full of buttons," he told me, his face a mask of rage and pain. "She'd gotten hungry. My bride."

Ann lived for nine years after she was diagnosed, but after three she was gone, her identity stolen. Only in retrospect would Lee understand how close he came to becoming gone himself.

After that first job as an assistant principal, Lee rose through the ranks of Connecticut administrators. He went back to school part-time and completed his masters in education and served seventeen years in administration before landing his first appointment as a superintendent of schools. By then things had gotten a little easier financially. They'd borrowed money from Ann's parents, other money from the bank, and cashed in a paid-up life insurance policy in order to make a down payment on their first home, a modest cape, and later, as the family grew, moved to a larger house in North Haven.

Once the children were old enough to attend school, Ann returned to part-time work. She organized the distribution of flu vaccines for North Haven, and later worked in a college admissions office. Caring, scrupulously honest, and wonderfully straightforward, she excelled in meeting people and helping them to solve their problems, large and small. But she was always home in time to meet the kids when they returned from school.

Their lives in Connecticut were rich and full, though Lee was beginning to experience the myriad headaches of being a superintendent of schools in Connecticut, whose average professional life expectancy was three years. Each administrator had to answer to and satisfy a school board of eight members who, as Lee put it, usually couldn't agree on a color. His last board in Connecticut was a particularly contentious group. They split right down the middle on every issue put before them, including, finally, whether to renew Lee's contract.

Lee wasn't one to walk away from a fight, but it occurred to him that here was a wonderful opportunity to act unilaterally, something administrators almost never get to do. He resigned and the following year accepted a superintendency in Winslow, Maine, where he would serve for seventeen years until he retired. He and Ann bought a house with several lovely acres of land in rural Vassalboro. They had four children by then. Only Maury, the youngest, was still in high school. Bruce, Kathy, and Suzanne were grown and beginning adult lives and families of their own as far away as California.

Lee and Ann had good reason to be proud not just of what they'd done but how they'd done it. And they had every reason to be optimistic about the future, until the afternoon the funny thing happened and Ann couldn't remember how to get home.

Eventually, no matter how much you might wish it otherwise, it all comes down to when. The first when is, When do I need help? and the answer is: Sooner than you think. If you're a man like Lee Duff, optimistic and resourceful by nature and training, and if you've spent most of your adult life problem-solving and believing that problems can be solved, your character strengths now turn on you the way rogue cells turn on the body whose immune system has been compromised.

You think that you can do this job. You think that it's your job to do, not someone else's. You try and you keep trying. Caregivers for people with terminal diseases know that in the end they will lose their loved one. What's not so apparent is that, without proper support, there's a good chance that the caregiver will be lost as well. Each eventually "goes into a hole," is the way Lee puts it. But you don't always recognize where you are.

In a couple of ways Lee was fortunate. He had invested wisely and was earning enough to hire secondary caregivers. Even with all this, the financial strain of a long-term disease can be breathtaking. Without it, you can lose everything. Lee estimates that Anne's care, from beginning to end, cost about a quarter of a million dollars, and that it'd be closer to twice that today. He was also fortunate to have a demanding job that required his full focus. Lee was someone whose competence and vision other people depended upon.

Also, many of the people he worked with understood what he was going through, and that helped enormously. But leaving Ann each morning to go to work made him feel both guilty and ashamed. She didn't understand where he was going or why he had to leave or why she couldn't go with him.

And not all of the people he hired to help out were well-suited to the task. Seeing that their patient was becoming child-like, they tried to engage Ann with games and activities. Eventually, though, Lee found the perfect secondary caregiver, a lovely woman named Desirae who worked for an agency called Helping Hands. She was young and recently married and Ann liked her. When Desirae got pregnant Lee assumed he'd have to start looking again, but when Desirae had her baby, Ann immediately bonded with the child, cuddling her at first, and then, when she started to toddle, following her around the house. Desirae went from part-time to full, and sometimes when Lee arrived home later than expected, the two of them would drop with exhaustion. "I'm thinking of adopting you," he told her.

Difficult though that first *when* is to gauge, the second is even harder, more soul-destroying. Lee knew that eventually he would have to put Ann in a nursing home. Though she was no longer really Ann, the body that had once housed Ann's mind, her memory, her spirit, soldiered on and would so continue for years. But knowing that something must be done is not the same as knowing when to do it. You discover it's possible to look into nursing homes and to decide, quite rationally, which will be the best "when the time comes," even as you tell yourself that you would never, ever do that. And even as you tell yourself that a nursing home is not an option, you worry there won't be a space when the time comes to do what you've sworn you'd never do. And then, unexpectedly, you *do* know. *When* arrives and it trails even more guilt. The only thing that keeps the guilt at bay, at least a little, is your exhaustion. The truest thing you know is that after all these hours and weeks and months and years, you're simply too tired to continue.

In Lee's case the decision of where to place Ann was made a little easier by the fact that her mother was still alive. She called Lee and begged him to put Ann in the home in Houlton. That way she could visit her daughter every day. Ann's mother was in her eighties now, and visiting Ann regularly in Vassalboro was impossible. Naturally, Lee was conflicted. Houlton was a three-hour drive, and if it meant that Ann's mother could visit her daughter more regularly, it also meant that Lee would be able to do so less often. Worse, there were conflicting symbolisms. If Ann went to Houlton, she'd be placed in the very facility where her father had been admitted during the final stages of his own Alzheimer's, a symmetry almost too cruel to contemplate. On the other hand, what geometric shape is more reassuring than a circle? What would be better than for Ann to end her days where she'd begun them? It was Lee's doctor who urged him to consider another possible benefit. Lee himself was spent, well beyond exhaustion. Placing Ann in Houlton might just save his life.

In addition to being blessed with a demanding job and some financial wherewithal, Lee was also blessed in the children he and Ann had raised. When the time came, all four kids returned home to help Lee take their mother north. They took two cars and arrived at the nursing home late in the afternoon. The staff advised them to make as little of the transition as possible, for their own sake, yes, but more importantly Ann's and the family's as well. They would be welcome to visit whenever they wanted, but today they should simply kiss Ann goodbye and leave. For Kathy and Suzanne, that proved impossible. They had to stay with their mother, at least for a while.

What was Lee feeling? An emptiness so profound he wouldn't have believed it possible. Guilt like an anvil. And always, these days, the exhaustion. But also something new, something so foreign, so alien and insidious he didn't immediately recognize it for what it was. Even surrounded by his children, Lee realized that he simply didn't want to live anymore.

Getting behind the wheel for the long drive home, he was again that ten-year-old boy driving a tractor in the dark, assigned a task that was too great for him (he can't reverse it, he can't control it, she's gone). Had he tried? Had he kept trying? At that moment he couldn't have said. All he knew was that he was returning home, the job undone, something his father had told him long ago that you simply did not do.

That was the bottom. It lasted a while but not forever. Despair, like a car thief, had paid him a visit, gained entry, then looked around, glimpsed his host's great reservoir of strength and optimism, and thought to himself, why struggle when the next vehicle was probably unlocked, unprotected, an invitation. This one would be nothing but trouble.

For the next three years Lee visited Ann in Houlton, every other week at first, then once a month. Sometimes one of the kids would go with him, but they all came to the same reluctant understanding—Ann never knew. The visits were known only to the visitors, though, as Lee put it, "She was still there, still mine."

And so it continued until Ann's body finally succumbed, long years after her spirit had fled. Lee and his younger son Maury were there when it happened, saw Ann's features, so long frozen in pain and perplexity, relax in the moment of release, saw the wife and mother they'd known in life returned to them now in death, angelic. The entire family gathered for a memorial service in Houlton, after which Ann's ashes were scattered on Nickerson Lake, a remote and beautiful spot accessible only by boat or on foot, where she'd spent summers as a child. The family has a rustic cottage there, which Lee now tends, spring and fall, one of his myriad responsibilities, at least half of which he's taken on since he retired, since Ann's death.

Perhaps the most important of these new duties is that he's now president of the board of the Hospice Volunteers of Waterville Area (HVWA). Dale Marie Clark, who directs the program and knew both Lee and Ann, recruited him several years ago. He also volunteers with Alzheimer's patients and caregivers. He knows what the latter, especially, are going through.

Part of what makes his story so remarkable, I think, is that at the time he could have used its services, he had no idea that hospice provided such a wide range of them, including Alzheimer's care and counseling. He freely acknowledges how lucky he was to have four loving children, friends, and a demanding job to help him through his and Ann's long ordeal. But he also knows how close he came to losing everything anyway.

What he needed, though he didn't know it at the time, was to talk to someone who'd gone through what he was experiencing, someone who could say, "Here's something that worked for me," or, "Here's something to watch out for." And, perhaps most importantly,

"This happened to me too. I didn't think I'd live through it, but here I am."

And Lee is still here. Every now and then we play racquetball, and he still wants me to understand who my ass belongs to (not me). "Trombones!" he announces when he takes the lead at seven to six, and then serves before I'm ready. "People think Hospice is about death," he says, "but they're wrong. It's about life."

Lee is remarried now, to a lovely woman named Barbara, who has a teenage daughter. They are a family. His present happiness is in no way rooted in forgetfulness. Time has afforded him a kind of clarity. He knows now what exhaustion and despair had blinded him to earlier—that he did everything he could, fulfilled every promise, every duty demanded by love and faith. He knows that he couldn't have done anything more without losing himself in the bargain, and knows that neither Ann nor his love and devotion to her demanded that sacrifice.

Still, Ann is never far from his thoughts, nor is the good life they created for themselves and their children. Sometimes he slips up and calls Barbara "Ann," which embarrasses him (who is not embarrassed when the mind plays its small tricks?). Barbara, of course, understands (*You know who you are!*). They have a full, busy life. At the end of the long interview that was the basis of this story, Lee consulted his watch, saw that we'd run long, and quickly got to his feet. He'd love to give me more time, he said, but he was overdue for one meeting and had another after that. There were problems looming and he wasn't sure he had the solutions. But never mind. He'd try something. If that didn't work, he'd try something else. A man after my own heart.

"You live 'til you die," he reminds me as we shake hands.

And that's how we leave it.

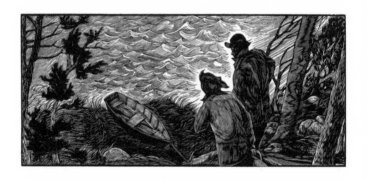

STAN SPOORS AND THE HORNBOOK OF THE HEART

Wesley McNair

> *"Do you not see how necessary a world of pain and troubles is to school an intelligence and make it a soul?*
>
> *. . . . I will call the human heart the hornbook used in that school."*
>
> —John Keats

In the first anger management workshop Stan Spoors led as a volunteer at Camp Ray of Hope, the annual Hospice retreat held in Winthrop, Maine, he got the idea of breaking plates. He and others on the staff hung plastic tarps from floor to ceiling on one side of the utility room where workshops are held, and twenty participants, all of whom had experienced the death of a family member, took turns breaking plates and bowls against the wall. Before they started, Stan gave them a few instructions. Each time they lifted a plate from the stack to break it, he says, they had to envision the person or thing that made them angry about the death, then address the object of their anger in any way they saw fit. "Rage is a natural part of the grieving process," he explains, "but people often get stuck in the rage. I wanted to give them a method of dealing with the anger they felt without hurting themselves or anybody else."

Out of the corner of his eye while the workshop participants were stepping up one by one to put on safety glasses and break dishes, Stan saw a woman standing in a corner near the door taking it all in, the same woman staff members had seen at the edges of group activities earlier in the day. "Her husband had just committed suicide and left her with two children, and we could see she was very troubled about that," Stan recalls. "We all thought she was going to bolt," he adds. But the woman by the door did not leave. She waited until the rest of the participants were done, then walked carefully across the shards of crockery to ask him if she could break some dishes, too. She couldn't do it in front of everyone else, she told him, so Stan cleared the room, gave her a stack of plates, and she started in. "She was real quiet at first," Stan remembers. "Gradually she began to say things like, 'How could you leave us alone like this?' and 'Look what you did to the kids.' She must have broken three or four dozen dishes before she came to the last one."

But for some reason the woman could not break that last plate. She held it in her hand and stared at it for a minute, then asked Stan if she could take it outside and pitch it into the nearby lake. If she wasn't able to break it, she told him, she could at least throw it away. They walked together along the wooded shore until she found an open place, then flung the plate as hard as she could out into the water. "When she turned back to me," he says, "she looked as though she might fall down, so I asked her, 'Can I give you a hug?' She put her arms out and completely collapsed, leaning against me for five or ten minutes. The anger and the tears just flowed out of her."

After the crying stopped, she told him the story of why she couldn't break the last plate. It reminded her, she said, of the china she and her husband had bought for their new home just before he committed suicide. All she wanted to do when she found he had taken his own life and left her behind was to break that china, she added, but destroying it meant also doing away with the dream of their shared life in the new home. She could not smash the last plate against the wall in Stan's workshop any more than she could bear to break the china. Throwing the plate into the lake instead, she was both getting rid of it and preserving it.

A Healing Touch

The next morning at breakfast when the woman sought Stan out to thank him, her mood was so much better, he hardly recognized her. "I want you to know you're the reason I was able to smile this morning when I got out of bed," she told him. Stan surprised her by thanking her back. "Every year at camp," he said, "it turns out there is one person I'm here for, above and beyond all the others. I'm grateful to you for being that person."

Listening to Stan Spoors relate his anecdote about the woman and the plates while I sit with him at the Hospice Community Center in Waterville, I understand why she opened up to him, just as parents and spouses and teenagers by the dozens have done since he started his hospice work several years ago. Stan is a tall man with over-the-collar gray hair, a full beard and an alert, generous face. When you talk with him, you have the sense he is really listening to what you have to say, and he has a ready and sympathetic laugh. His co-workers are no less drawn to him than the bereaved people he counsels. "He has a feeling for others that's deep in his being—in his soul," explains Dale Marie Clark, Executive Director of Hospice Volunteers at the Center. What he brings to the camp community each year, she says, is not only his gift of compassion, but also a kind of joy.

A sure sign of that joy is Lester Flatlander, the comic character Stan has created to entertain those who attend the camp's No-Talent Talent Show on Saturday nights. Wearing a worn hat and disheveled clothes, Stan takes the stage to play Lester, a womanizing sage "from away," opposite Effie Spitfire, his girlfriend and nemesis, who appears from the wings just as Lester begins to play "Devil Woman" on his guitar. "I don't want to stay/I want to get away," he intones, "Woman, let go of my arm"—which is exactly the moment when Effie begins to yank on Lester's sleeve. The audience, Stan says, just loves it. He follows it up at the late-night campfire by playing tunes participants request on his guitar accompanied by other musicians, and on Sunday, at the retreat's memorial service, he performs electronic music on his keyboard. His signature offering is "Tears in Heaven." The simple and moving lyrics of this song, composed by Eric Clapton after the death of his young son, apply to anyone who grieves the loss of a loved one, and when Stan sings it, there is hardly a dry eye in the house.

I gradually realize as our conversation deepens that the authority Stan brings to the Clapton song at the Sunday service, and to all of his work for hospice, comes from his own experience with tears and grieving. That experience began on another Sunday long ago, when he was just seven years old. His family was getting ready to go to church at their home in rural Michigan, he says, when the next-door neighbor, a fundamentalist Christian like his father, began to pound on the front door, shouting about the sinful nature of what the family's dog Duke, Stan's constant companion, was doing right on the lawn. "My father stepped outside the house to find Duke copulating with the neighbor's dog, and he was outraged. So he went back inside and got his sixteen-gauge shotgun, and while my brother and I watched from the doorway, he walked straight out to the dogs and shot Duke in the head."

That same year Stan's mother discovered that his father—who, despite his religious preachings, had often been unfaithful to her—was seeing still another woman. This time she decided to leave him, but not before she confronted the woman and listed all his lies and infidelities. When she came home to tell her husband what she had done and pack her bags, he began to pick up household objects and hurl them against the wall, turning into what Stan calls "the monster in the house." He broke every piece of furniture, and when he was finished, he tore the framed pictures and mirrors from their nails and broke them. Then he turned to the dishes. "Not a plate in our house was unbroken," Stan says. Meanwhile, Stan stood outside all alone (he does not remember where his brothers were), forgotten by his parents. Sensing that his mother, with whom he had a special bond, would soon come out with her packed bags, he went to the car and pulled out a spark-plug wire. "That didn't stop her," he says. "Even though the engine didn't sound so good, my mother, my protector, drove off leaving me in a cloud of dust. So I ran away myself and hid out for a long time at the farm across the road."

"Eventually, my father and mother reconciled," Stan says, taking a deep breath and shaking his head, "but they should have gone their separate ways right then." He doesn't recall the details of the reconciliation; in fact, he remembers little from his childhood, which is a complete blank, he says, except for those two traumatic events when he was seven. At eighteen, after continuous struggles with his father, he moved out of the family house in Grand Haven, ending up in the city of Grand Rapids. There, with few possessions besides his beloved guitar, he lived on the streets and began using recreational drugs, his situation among the homeless an echo of the homelessness he had felt even as he lived under his parents' roof.

"Everyone liked me when I was using LSD, my drug of choice," he remembers, "but when I wasn't high, I was miserable and angry a lot of the time, even violent. I didn't hurt anybody, but I beat up a lot of walls"—which is to say, Stan turned the anger he felt on himself. In calmer hours, he composed music by ear on his guitar, and he became known among his street friends for a particular song whose refrain about the chains that bound him referred to the traumas of his early home life. He not only memorized the lyrics of this song; he wrote them down in poetic form and kept them with him for years afterward as a kind of talisman, a charm against the emotional problems that troubled him.

Not long after Stan arrived in Grand Rapids in the early '70s, he began dating Sandra Samelot, a young woman he met there, and when she got pregnant, the two of them married and moved into a run-down apartment that his wife, employed at the local hospital, put up the money for. Stan had great plans for renovating the place, but the plans never materialized. His marriage, which officially lasted two years, was actually over in three months. By the time his son Steven was born, Stan had already left his wife and she was living with her mother. "After a point, I just never went home," Stan recalls. "I returned to my street life and began chasing women. I see, looking back," he says, "that I didn't go home because I was terrified of being the kind of father my own father was. Under the surface, I was still the seven-year-old kid who ran away and hid from the monster in the house. Ironically, even though I didn't want to turn into my father, I was becoming just like him."

Married and divorced at the age of twenty-one, he moved back to Grand Haven, getting a job as a forklift operator in an automobile parts plant and putting his street life behind him. "Things seemed to be going pretty well," Stan says, "until one day at work when the buzzer went off to announce the morning break. I tried to get down from the forklift and my legs wouldn't work." An ambulance came and took him to the hospital, where doctors x-rayed and tested him for a week trying to find out what was wrong. Unable to discover any physical reason for the dysfunction, they finally transferred him to a hospital with a behavior modification unit. After over a month of counseling there, Stan's psychiatrist determined that his illness was psychosomatic, caused by the two traumas he had experienced as a boy and perhaps by other childhood events unrecovered by memory.

It would be comforting to report that Stan discovered through his dysfunction the relationship between his past and his failures in the present, shedding the chains that bound him. But the important insights in life seldom come easily. What happened instead was that he remarried, and amidst new hopes of making a home, began to repeat his old mistakes. Eventually he married again, to Pamela Osborne, becoming the father of a second child, his daughter Lisa. Amidst new hopes of making a home, Stan began to repeat his old mistakes. Shortly after Lisa was born in 1983, the marriage broke up, a casualty of Stan's absences and infidelities. Six years later, he was on to marriage number three.

Yet now he was well into his thirties, and his attitude had taken a dramatic turn. "For one thing, I was head-over-heels in love," he explains. "But beyond that, I was at last ready to be a husband and change my ways." This time, there was no more running around and no more running away from home. If any problems surfaced in his relationship with the third Mrs. Spoors, nee Velcie Hickman, he stood ready to take the blame for them. "As far as I was concerned, she could do no wrong. Whenever she seemed disappointed, I did everything I could to please her."

Stan's new attitude went a great way toward preserving the marriage. As it turned out, his wife was often angry with him and susceptible to fits of jealous rage. She began to watch the clock at the end of his work day at the IRS office, and if he arrived home only minutes late, she accused him of having an affair. Once after work, he paused to show off a new car they had bought to a fellow employee and got home to discover her throwing all his belongings out the door of their apartment. Before he got married to his new wife, her own sister, a co-worker at the IRS, had warned him she was bound to be trouble, and his wife's irrational behavior suggested the sister was right. Still, Stan was undeterred. "I would have made a contract with the devil to stay in that marriage," he says. Lester Flatlander had met his Effie Spitfire.

Within a year his wife was pregnant with their child, and Stan was euphoric. "I was not only ready to be a husband, come what may," he explains, "I was ready to be a father. I felt I'd been given a chance to make up for all the mistakes I'd made."

An amniocentesis their doctor performed on his wife determined the baby was normal and healthy, and ultrasound pictures showed he was a boy. As the birth date neared, the couple spent hours over lists of baby names, finally settling on "Justin Scott." He made a dot-matrix picture of a baby bearing his son's name and taped it to the cassette case he took to work. "I'd put the case right on my desk with the picture facing out so everybody passing by could see it," he says. He and his wife went shopping for Justin, buying him a deluxe playpen and an array of toys. And on the day the baby arrived, after an arduous birth, Stan phoned everyone in his family—even his father, whom he almost never called—to tell them the news.

But by the time he made those phone calls, Stan had become deeply apprehensive about his son. For one thing, Justin was born seven weeks before his due date in late November 1990, and worse still, his heart had stopped; a team of doctors and nurses had to work on him with defribrillator paddles to start it beating again.

Detecting a heart murmur, the doctors investigated further, discovering another serious problem. Despite the earlier prognosis that Justin would be normal and healthy, he had a hole through all four chambers of his heart. Surgery could correct the problem, the doctors said, but only after Justin was six months old. "Every day after that there seemed to be something new to deal with," Stan says. "First they said four cervical vertebrae were missing, preventing Justin from turning his head to the left. Then they said he had a partial cleft pallette, which meant he couldn't suck and feeding had to be done with a syringe. Then they told us his intestines were malrotated, so he had to be fed small amounts every two hours around the clock." Finally doctors informed Stan and his wife that Justin had developed only thirty percent of his cerebral cortex. As the bad news about Justin's condition unfolded, Stan says, "my whole world began to collapse."

Just before Thanksgiving, however, when Justin was over a month old, the doctors agreed to release him to the care of his parents, and as Stan spent time at home with his son, his spirits began to lift. "To see him smile, you would never have guessed he had all those problems they talked about," he recalls. "He seemed like any other baby, except unlike most babies, he never cried—only once, when he had his first bath." Gradually, Stan came to think of Justin's special needs as challenges rather than burdens. Anyway, he was smitten. "I was so pleased to have him home," he says, "I couldn't stand myself. I even took him to work with me one day. I must have shown him to all 1200 employees at the IRS."

The time Stan enjoyed most with Justin, though, was the early morning when he fed him with the syringe. His wife asleep, Stan would make a fire just for his son and himself in the fireplace. "That was our time," Stan remembers. "While I split kindling for the fire, I'd be showing him how to do it. I'd open one hand and tell him, 'These are fingers. You're not supposed to cut these.' Sometimes I held up something red or green to teach him his colors. I'd tell him about the bees and the grasshoppers, or sing him dirty sailor ditties."

Imagine Stan's misery, then, when he was suddenly prevented from seeing Justin at all. His wife, in a new round of jealousy and paranoia, called him at work after the Thanksgiving holiday to discover he was late returning from lunch. When he called her back, worn out by conflicts with her, she was in the midst of throwing his possessions out the door again, and so angry that he went home to try and talk her down. There, he found Justin all alone on the couch without blankets or his heart monitor, and nothing to prevent him from falling on the floor. Now it was Stan's turn to be upset, and he was furious.

"My son," he told her, "needs better care than that." He loaded up his belongings in his truck, then went back to get Justin and take him away. But by that time his wife had called up both her father and the police, and her father met him at the door.. Stan soon found himself in court, trying to get custody of Justin before a judge, though to no avail.

For three weeks afterward he could only learn about Justin's welfare through his wife's sister at work. Then, on the last day of December, a doctor telephoned him. Justin had been admitted to the emergency room with pneumonia, he said, and was in serious condition. Stan rushed to the hospital and began an anxious vigil of nine days and nights, able to visit Justin for just ten minutes of every hour in intensive care, where he lay under a respirator. As it turned out, his son was never to leave the intensive care unit. On January 9, 1991, at three months of age, Justin died.

On the very day of Justin's funeral, Stan remembers, his wife told him she wanted a divorce. After everyone left the funeral and he was all by himself, he says, he felt more alone than he had ever been. Through all the missed connections and the detours of his life, Stan Spoors had really been driven by one basic thing: the wish for a family that would love him and that he could love in return. But events from past to present seemed to have conspired against that wish, leaving him with nothing to show for it. After Justin's passing and his wife's departure, he was a little like the bereft woman by the lake at Camp Ray of Hope holding her last plate, the emblem of a lost home life. The difference was that for Stan, there was no one around to reach out to in his despair.

Left to his own devices, he turned to poetry, just as he had turned to song lyrics years before in a troubled period, writing three poems about Justin through his tears, then rereading the words he had written to assuage his pain. In one of the poems, which he has kept to this day, he remembers the "feedings in the middle of the night" and his "chats" with Justin by the fire. In another, he recalls Justin's smile that brought pleasure to those around him. In a third, he longs to be with Justin in heaven so he can cradle him in his arms. But no matter how hard Stan worked on the poems or how often he returned to them, they didn't provide the solace he was desperate for.

In November of 1991, when his divorce was finalized, he began to suffer from severe migraine headaches, and by January, the month of Justin's death a year earlier, he was drawn into a spiral of depression that pills could not relieve. One day at work, "just wanting to end the pain," as Stan puts it, he downed a whole bottle of anti-depressants. He didn't regain consciousness for nearly a week. When he finally woke up, he was in the psych ward at the hospital, surprised to find himself in restraints. He had been violent with the staff, a nurse told him.

Like Stan Spoors, I myself have turned to poetry for solace, sometimes writing my own poems, sometimes memorizing the lines of other poets to calm myself in troubled moments. One poem I have by heart is John Keats's "When I Have Fears That I May Cease To Be," a great cry of the spirit against the finality of death. Another is Emily Dickinson's poem 419. In this verse Dickinson likens the darkest periods of our existence to walking without a path on a moonless and starless night—an evening, as she calls it, "of the Brain." For those who have experienced such an evening, she suggests, the darkness never really lifts; yet they can learn to walk in it if they can find the courage. "The Bravest," she says,

– grope a little –
And sometimes hit a Tree
Directly in the Forehead –
But as they learn to see –
Either the darkness alters –

Or something in the sight
Adjusts itself to Midnight –
And life steps almost straight.

The description Dale Clark recently gave me of
what happens to a family member following the death
of a loved one recalls Dickinson's poem. "Everything
they've believed in has been stripped from them, and
suddenly they're all alone, forced to see the world in a
different way." Recovering, she says, is not so much a
matter of getting over the loss as learning to live with
it, and with the reality that "anything can be taken
from them at any time."

Stan Spoors' first lessons in how to walk in the
dark came from meetings of The Compassionate
Friends, the national organization specializing in help
for bereaved parents. Put in touch with the local chapter of The Compassionate Friends by a psychologist at
the hospital, he began to listen to the stories of others
who had lost children. "Seeing how other people got
through their pain," he explains, "I would feel a spark
of hope. Then it would go out. I lived my life in minutes, managing to get through one minute, and telling
myself that maybe now I could live through the next
one." He went to more meetings; gradually he began to

complete whole days without second-guessing them; then he was able to complete a week.

And throughout the period of what Stan calls his healing, there were stories, not only the ones other grief-stricken family members told him about their experiences, but the one he told them about his own loss and despair. As meetings went on and new people joined Stan's counseling group, he told his personal story over and over. "We know that expressing thoughts and feelings is part of the healing process," says one of the principals of the Compassionate Friends. "We need not walk alone," declares their credo. Telling his story to audiences who listened with genuine concern, Stan took his first steps in the company of others.

In a culture like ours, which tends to gloss over tragedy and insist on quick fixes, the time it takes a heart to mend after the death of a family member may seem impossibly slow. Stan's recovery from Justin's death, complicated by other family traumas, began in late 1991 and was still in progress in 1996. During that year he was on a week-long fishing trip, and his brother Doug played an Eric Clapton CD that included the song "Tears in Heaven." In the haunting and moving lyrics of this song, Clapton, accompanying himself on accoustic guitar, tells his own story of bereavement following his son's accidental death. He begins by imagining an encounter with his son in heaven:

Would you know my name
If I saw you in heaven?
Would it be the same
If I saw you in heaven?

Those opening questions are followed later on by two others:

Would you hold my hand
If I saw you in heaven?
Would you help me stand
If I saw you in heaven?

In the chorus of the song the father cries out in sorrow, longing to be with his child again:

Time can break your heart
Have you beggin' please, beggin' please...

"I had never heard of Clapton before, but this song had an immediate impact on me," Stan says.

"I asked Doug to play it again. I played it every time I got the chance, all week long." A guitarist and singer who had lost a son himself, Stan had suddenly found an ally.

Like Clapton, Stan had also written a poem about meeting his son in heaven. But the encounter in the Clapton song was different. It was not a wish-fulfillment dream that put aside life on earth, as Stan's poem had done, but an acceptance of earthly life, however difficult that acceptance might be in the face of the child's death. So in his second verse, Clapton sings:

I'll find my way
Through night and day
'Cause I know I just can't stay
Here in heaven.

While there is sorrow in the song's concluding verse, there is also affirmation, because it describes a reconciliation with the son's death and the end of tears.

Beyond the door
There's peace I'm sure,
And I know there'll be no more
Tears in heaven.

Stan was amazed that Eric Clapton could get through "Tears in Heaven" without breaking down— that he could express such deep feelings about his son's death and hold himself apart from them at the same time. As he played the track over and over, Stan was no doubt relearning from his fellow song-writer and guitarist the power of creative expression to make order out of life's confusion. But he was also learning that like Clapton, he needed to accept the death of his son and enter more fully into his life on earth, imperfect as that life might seem.

As it happened, Stan was not only accompanied by his brother Doug on the week of his fishing trip, but by his father. In fact, his whole purpose on the trip was to make peace with his father. To Stan, the time seemed right for reconciliation. The enormity of Justin's death had made the problems his father caused years before seem small by comparison. Besides, Stan had realized long since that he had made mistakes of his own. His father, for his part, had just suffered a life-threatening bout of kidney cancer, and now felt compelled to make things right with his son.

"During that trip he was a different man," Stan explains. "Earlier on, when I called him about Justin's death, he told me all my problems would go away if I joined the church. But now when I talked about Justin, he put aside the religious stuff and really wanted to know how I was doing. Mostly, though," he adds, "we weren't being serious at all. The three of us just made jokes back and forth and enjoyed each other's company. It was a terrific week. I felt for the first time since Justin's funeral that I wasn't living in isolation—that there were people in the world who really cared about me." It is likely that the Eric Clapton song Stan played over and over helped him reach out to his father during the family retreat. For the song's message of acceptance was as important to Stan's relationship with his father as it was to his relationship with his lost son.

Stan's discovery of "Tears in Heaven" and the family closeness he found on the fishing trip marked a turning point in his healing. Over time, his reconciliation with his father led him to reach out to others he had left behind in the past—his first wife, for instance, and his daughter and first son. Moreover, he began to undertake the hospice work he does today, editing a newsletter for The Compassionate Friends, in which he wrote a column of stories about the bereaved, then starting an online chat room on a Web site called "The Forties" for people his age who had suffered the death of a loved one.

A Healing Touch

Telling stories about the losses of others and counseling them over the Internet had a profound effect on Stan's healing. "I survived," he recalls, "by helping others to survive."

Through his online work he met his current partner, Gloria, who ran the "Forties" website. A bereaved parent like him, Gloria helped with the counseling. It did not matter that he had no formal training for his work. He "used hard knocks" as his guide, relying on the hornbook of the heart, to use the metaphor of the poet John Keats, and what the hornbook had taught him. Stan had, he says, just two goals. The first was getting the chat room visitors to talk about their personal experience, just as he had done, in an atmosphere of understanding, and the second was giving them hope that they could find their way through their desolation. What he wanted was what he wants today for those he counsels in hospice: to see that something good can come from their situation. "I tell them they can make a success out of their tragedy," he says. "I'm always thrilled when I watch them take that first step forward."

For like Emily Dickinson, who described the attempt to walk in spite of darkness, and like John Keats, who wrote about the uses of suffering, Stan has come to realize that extremes of emotional distress can lead to a new state of awareness. "It reshapes who you are," he says. When he started out in his twenties, he explains, he cared mainly about his own problems. But the depression and grief he experienced following Justin's death gave him a sympathy for the burdens others carry and a feeling that "the best help is offering help to somebody else."

Moving to Maine to be with Gloria in March of 2000, he founded the state's second chapter of The Compassionate Friends, in Dover-Foxcroft. Then he became a bereavement counselor at Dover-Foxcroft's Pine Tree Hospice. His activity for the bereaved culminated at the statewide Hospice retreat Camp Ray of Hope, in Winthrop, where he transformed his whole life experience into the work of compassion, from the breaking of plates in his anger management workshops, to fending off the attacks of Effie Spitfire as Lester Flatlander on Saturday nights, to offering his own arrangement of "Tears in Heaven" on Sundays, always singing the Clapton song especially for Justin, whose memory, Stan says, inspired everything he did at the camp. Finally, after all the difficulties in Stan Spoors' life, a happy ending.

At least that's what I'm thinking when I arrive at the Hospice Center for a follow-up conversation with Stan, ready to put the finishing touches on my article about him. "So," I say to him with a smile, recalling the account of his fortunate landing in Maine and the hospice work he took up here—"all's well that ends well, right?"

But Stan corrects me. All did not end well. After that happy moment in his life, things started to go wrong for him once more. His relationship with Gloria suffered a bad turn, and a break-up with her seemed all but inevitable. Then his father's second wife called from Michigan with the news that his father was seriously ill and in the hospital. He gathered up all his belongings, said goodbye to Gloria, and flew to Michigan, concerned about his father and despondent about the prospect of looking for a home all over again.

When he got to the hospital and found his father had terminal cancer, his concern turned to stress about the role he now faced as a caregiver. On disability retirement from the IRS, he was the son best able to help during his father's final days. Still, Stan remembered the desolation of his last days with Justin, and he did not know if he was strong enough to repeat the experience.

Yet here, in the midst of Stan's anxiety and sorrow, is where the happy ending begins. It turned out that his long experience with hospice work had prepared him for this death, not only informing him about the stages his father went through during the eight months of his dying, but also helping him cope with his own bereavement during the terminal illness. Moreover, his father was entirely at ease with his situation, and more open with Stan than he had ever been. "We could talk about anything," Stan says. When he brought up the subject of his dog Duke, whose death he had never properly grieved, tears came to his father's eyes: "I've felt bad about that ever since it happened," he said. Revisiting the event became a way for the two of them to grieve for the long-lost dog together. Stan was surprised to discover that his other early trauma, the breaking of household furniture and plates, was also an old source of guilt for his father, and moreover, that the old man had been upset all through the period of their estrangement. As he listened to his father confess his remorse, the last vestige of the chains Stan had written about in a song lyric years before disappeared. "I told him, 'Dad, the bottom line is, you did the best you could with the resources you had.'" After his father was released from the hospital for home care, they were with each other constantly. Sometimes they did wood-carving in his father's basement workshop; sometimes they just sat in the kitchen drinking coffee and talking about whatever came up. "It didn't really matter what we were doing," Stan recalls, "we were just content to be together. I had never felt so close to my father. I like to think my being there with him had a lot to do with his serenity at the time of his death."

As for ceasing the relationship with Gloria, which seemed unavoidable when Stan flew to Michigan, that was not to be. She was on the phone with him from Maine almost every day, checking in. Often their conversation turned to what went wrong between them, and they discovered they had expectations of each other that were unrealistic. Eventually they found themselves making commitments to each other about the things they would and wouldn't do when they got back together in Maine. A few weeks after his father's death, Stan returned to Gloria, having taken vows with a mate that were based on reality, rather than wishes, for the first time in his life. "In March the two of us were together for seven years," he declares with a grin. "I've broken my own record. And I'm looking forward to eight and nine and ten years after that."

For Stan Spoors has at last found his true home, which includes not only the house he shares with Gloria, but also the Hospice Community Center, where he has come to sit with me and tell his story, and Camp Ray of Hope, the retreat that the center sponsors. At the camp, he is not called Stan, but "Stosh," an old family nickname, and he thinks of the people there as "my family." They are, after all, kindred spirits. Like him, many have been broken by loss and despair, and like him, others have been moved to help the broken ones put themselves back together. If they knew his long journey of tragedy, courage, and hope, they would see why it is that he brings such a depth of understanding to his work there, giving it his whole heart.

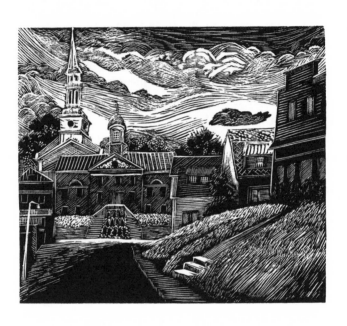

THE QUILT PEOPLE
Susan Sterling

> *No one is as capable of gratitude as one who has emerged*
> *from the kingdom of night. We know that every moment*
> *is a moment of grace, every hour an offering; not to share*
> *them would mean to betray them. Our lives no longer belong*
> *to us alone; they belong to all those who need us desperately.*
>
> Holocaust survivor Elie Wiesel
> (*quoted in Molly Fumia*, Safe Passage)

It's a startlingly beautiful Saturday afternoon in late September in central Maine, summer-like weather, the leaves just beginning to turn, the bereaved families at Camp Ray of Hope in shorts and T-shirts. On the pond, campers are fishing and paddling around in canoes. Just past the lodge, a young man leaps into the cold waters to swim.

In the camp dining hall, Sandra Kervin works with her sewing machine, surrounded by scraps of fabric and ribbons. She's leading a workshop for children and adults in making "memory pillows." Nearby, at another long table, children decorate white baseball hats with stickers and glitter markers.

A Healing Touch

On the walls behind Sandra hang three large quilts.

Late in the afternoon my husband stops by for a brief visit. He meets me at the lodge porch where I've just spent the afternoon leading journal workshops. Many of the participants have been young widows with children, and working with them, giving them a chance to write and talk about their grief, has been both exhilarating and heartbreaking. I pack up the leftover journals and pens, then take my husband back along the camp road so that he can see Sandra's family quilt, hanging in the dining hall. I've tried to describe this quilt to him before, but I've failed to evoke its beauty. A quilt made from her son's clothes, I said. His jeans, his fishing license, his car key, his baseball cap.

The hall is noisy with children's energy, but standing before the quilt, both of us fall quiet. Like my husband, I had a hard time visualizing Sandra's quilt before I saw it and did not imagine I would be so moved. After the deaths of my mother and younger sister, I tried to find my way along the path of grief with words, reading and writing. Sandra has stitched her way.

Images of a road, or a path, often appear when mourners talk about their experiences of loss. If grief is a journey, then the itinerary at its most heartening involves getting from here to there, from devastation to acceptance. By "there" I don't mean "closure," that deceptive term that suggests painful experiences can be shut away in a closet labeled "The Past." The journey is long and arduous, particularly when death is sudden or unexpected or violent. What one hopes for is the faith that life still has meaning. The path is highly individual and never clearly set out. It might most accurately be depicted with a related image, as a trail one makes oneself through a dark and lonely wood, hoping to glimpse a clearing.

Having found myself wandering in these dark woods—once as my mother lay dying from cancer, and eight years ago after the probable suicide of my younger sister—I listen with admiration and curiosity to the stories others tell me, sometimes with envy for the beliefs they've found or reaffirmed. Some stories, like that of Sandra Kervin and her family completely draw me in.

The Kervins' son Jarod died by suicide, a particularly devastating death. Though I find the phrase "survivor of suicide" misleading, suggesting someone who attempted suicide and didn't succeed, the term accurately evokes the trauma experienced by family and friends of the victim. Even if those who take their own lives feel they have no choice—indeed, they often tragically believe their family and friends will be better off without them—the death rarely appears inevitable to those left behind. Feelings of anger and guilt and abandonment invade them, as if love should or could have prevented what happened. Survivors relive, over and over, the last days and months, even years, before the suicide, seeing now the signs that were missed, which they believe they should have recognized.

As an added pain, the bereft suffer from the stigma that still shadows suicide. Often, family and friends will keep secret the reason for the death, or lie about it. For years, suicides were not allowed to be buried in the hallowed ground of a churchyard. My sister, who was fervently religious and a convert to the Eastern Orthodox Church, told her husband in a moment of despair the night before her death that she had thought of suicide, but she "didn't want to go to hell." Perhaps because of the stigma, relatives and friends often shy away from those bereaved by suicide or urge them to return quickly to life as it once was, as if the death had never happened.

After my mother's death, I came across these words of the French writer Albert Camus, which I placed on my desk and then returned to often after my sister died: "In the midst of winter, I finally learned that there was in me an invincible summer." The word "finally" reminds us that there is nothing sudden about recovering from a loss, no quick balm, no magical jolt back into life. Going on often begins with the smallest of gestures. First there is a taking, and then, after a long time, a giving and reaching out to others.

To begin, then, a real road: this one leading east from the central Maine town of Waterville, across the Kennebec River and up along the Sebasticook River to the small town of Albion. I first travel along this road one evening in late September 2006. It's dark, the early dark of fall in Maine, and I drive too far past the sharp bend in the road that Sandra has given me as a marker and arrive a little late. The Kervins' ranch house is set back from the road, and on the same piece of property, not a stone's throw from the front door, is the apartment—a converted garage—where eighteen-year-old Jarod Kervin was living when he shot himself on November 29, 1999.

A light is on outside the porch. I knock on the door, and when there's no response, let myself in. Sandra opens the door leading to the kitchen. "Ed and I must have fallen asleep watching TV," she explains apologetically. She takes me into the living room, which is lit by two large red candles. A television glows in the corner. There's a brief flurry while we establish whether I've inadvertently let out one of the two cats. (I haven't—the cats, one white, one calico, saunter in a few minutes later and stretch out on the living room rug.) Sandra telephones their younger son, Adam, who comes over from the apartment next door where he is now living. It was Adam, then twelve, who found Jarod's body there seven years ago. Now, like his older brother, he wants his independence but wants to remain close to his parents, as well, and it is a measure of how far they all have come since those dark days that the site of their tragedy has been transformed back into a young man's refuge.

The Kervins' daughter Lori and her 18-month-old baby, Ariel, also live in the main house with Sandra and Ed. On my first visit, the baby is asleep in a back room and Lori is at work. Lori was three weeks from her fifteenth birthday when her brother died. She lived on her own for a few years, but now she is back home, working evenings at Kohl's department store in Augusta, about half an hour away. Those evenings, Sandra and Ed take care of their granddaughter. During the day Sandra works at Inland Hospital in Waterville; Ed also works in Waterville, as the manager of the Dollar Tree.

I know Sandra from the Survivors of Suicide group, run by Hospice, that I co-facilitated in the fall of 2001, when she was a participant; two-and-a-half years later we led a similar group together. I have heard in some detail what we in Hospice call her "story"—that is, her version of Jarod's death and its aftermath—but I don't know Ed's or Adam's or Lori's stories, and I don't know much about their lives before 1999. So on my first visit in September, and then on a second visit in November, I ask the Kervins about their beginnings. I am curious about this family that has come through darkness and now describes their lives as in many ways blessed.

Sandra and Ed have not moved far from where they spent their childhoods. They both grew up in Waterville—Ed in an Irish-American family (his mother was half-Irish, half Franco-American), and Sandra in a Franco-American family. Sandra's mother died in 1988, eleven years before Jarod's death, when Jarod was seven. Ed's childhood stopped abruptly when he was quite young. His father died when he was seven, his mother when he was fourteen, after which he lived more or less on his own, finishing school and then joining the service. Since then, his two brothers, his uncle, his aunt, and a cousin have died, as well. Only his sister is still living. "At fifty-three, I'm the tail end of the family," he says. Still, none of these losses helped him with Jarod's death. "There was so much tucked away in the closet," he says of his growing up. "There was no one there for me when Mom was dying. I didn't want to open that door."

The couple met when they were both working at Inland Hospital in Waterville, Ed as a physical therapy assistant, Sandra in Central Services, where the hospital's instruments and needles are sterilized. They married in 1980. Eventually, Ed went into management and worked at Sam's Club and Service Merchandise in Augusta and then at the Dollar Tree in Waterville (where, at Adam's suggestion, I found journals for the participants in the Camp Ray of Hope workshops).

The Kervins describe Jarod's suicide as totally un-expected. They saw no warning signs, no previous struggle with depression. The night before his death, he spent the evening with the family in their living room, talking and watching television. When he didn't appear the next morning or answer the phone, Ed sent Adam over to check on him. Sandra had already left for work, and though she noticed the bedroom light was on in the apartment, not the living room light, which was unusual, and though Jarod didn't come out to say goodbye to her, as he almost always did, she didn't think much of it. Entering the apartment, Adam glimpsed his older brother's body, then ran back to the house, crying out, "There's a gun on the bed and blood everywhere!"

Ed ran next door, grabbed the gun out of his son's hand and threw it on the floor, then fled the apartment and called 911 and Sandra. The 911 dispatcher told him to go back in and check for a pulse, which he did, though he knew, from the stiffness of Jarod's hand where it had held the gun, that his son was already dead. "That was," he tells me, "maybe the hardest thing I had to do, going back in." A deputy from the Kennebec County Sheriff's Department arrived and called for backup. The police descended on the apartment, going through everything in their investigation. Though some communities now have trained teams who will go to a home where a suicide has taken place and assist the family, such help didn't exist in central Maine in 1999. The Kervins stood off to the side, in shock. "I have two words to describe the loss of my son," Ed tells me. "Total devastation."

The months after Jarod's death were chaotic. Ed doesn't remember much after the police came, except that for 47 of the next 48 hours he paced back and forth from one end of his living room to the other. He didn't know what to do. The police told him that Sandra shouldn't see the body, and so when she next saw Jarod, he was lying in an open casket at Veilleux's Funeral Home in Waterville, looking as he always had, except for a little swelling under the eyes. The workers at the funeral home did, according to Sandra, a fantastic job covering up the impact trauma. She had been surprised that the casket was open for the visiting hours, but it was important, she says, because a lot of people came to see him. The Kervins had been asked to bring Jarod's clothes, and Ed brought Jarod's new Reeboks. "My son will need these to walk through the Gates of Heaven," he told the funeral home director.

Ed and Sandra had sympathetic bosses who told them to take what time they needed to deal with the loss of their son. Still, the family all felt abandoned, unable to help each other, Jarod's death rending the fabric of their lives. In the chaotic months following, Sandra says she could see her family, once so close, falling apart, all of them grieving in different ways. But numbed with sorrow herself, she could only watch. All she and Ed could manage, it seemed, was to clean the house. The house was one thing they could control. They cleaned and cleaned. Fortunately, their really bad days seemed to alternate, so that when Sandra was having a difficult day, Ed was able to function, when he was flattened by sorrow, Sandra could take over. One of the managers where he works recently asked him how he got through that time. Ed ascribes his survival to his religious faith and Sandra: "I have an incredible spouse, and my faith runs very deep," he said.

The death, which came three weeks before Lori's fifteenth birthday, was especially disastrous for her. She felt she'd not only lost the brother she loved, but she'd also lost her parents, her whole family, the home she'd always known. The house was filled with pain and no longer felt safe to her. Her parents were not who they'd been. She ran away several times. The Kervins always brought her back home, troubled and angry.

Not too long after Jarod's death, someone gave Sandra the phone number of Dale Marie Clark, then director of bereavement services with the Waterville Hospice, but Sandra was skeptical, associating the organization with work with the terminally ill. "What for?" she asked herself. "He's already dead!" Eventually she called Dale, and at her suggestion, Sandra joined a Hospice group for grieving parents, but after two meetings she stopped going. It was just four months since Jarod's death, and she wasn't ready. Lori and Adam did, however, receive one-on-one bereavement counseling through Hospice, as did Sandra. The family limped along. Then, sometime in the summer, Dale came out to the house in Albion, appearing, as is so often mysteriously the case with her, at a moment of intense despair, as if knowledge of the family's descent into darkness traveled to her through the cosmos. She persuaded the family, in particular, Ed, to come to Camp Ray of Hope.

Another road then, this one both real and spiritual, appears in my conversation with the Kervins. The road leads to Camp Mechuawana, a Methodist camp on Lower Narrows Pond, near Winthrop, Maine, where Camp Ray of Hope has been held on the third weekend in September for the past eleven years.

I first experienced this road on a rainy Friday night in 1999, two months before Jarod's death and eight months after the death of my sister. The weather was damp and cold, and driving into the campgrounds with my daughter, I just wanted to turn back to our home in Waterville. All that winter and spring and summer, I'd felt a persistent grayness in my life. My husband, children, and friends had been wonderfully supportive (my daughter, then fifteen, had even offered to come with me that weekend). But being with other people could turn unexpectedly painful and bewildering, and I found it impossible to believe I would connect with anyone at the camp.

The Kervins felt the same apprehension when, the following September, they traveled that same road. Six years later, as we sit in their living room, the candles flickering and the cats sleeping on the floor between us, Ed describes their reluctance, similar to that of most first-time families, and their feelings of fear, uncertainty, and resistance. It was Sandra who dragged them all to Camp Ray of Hope, Ed says. He and Adam and Lori were just along for the ride. "What do I want to go to camp where everyone is sitting around crying?" he asked himself. "Then, when I got there, and we went into groups and people were laughing, I thought, I don't belong with these happy people!"

Sandra says she was numb most of the weekend. "Someone told me," she says, "that we had 'The Look.'" She hadn't a clue what this meant, but the next year, when she and Adam and Ed returned to Camp Ray of Hope for a second time, she recognized a blankness on the faces of the recently bereaved, and understood. What she saw were people who appeared haunted and bewildered, unable to fathom a world that would inflict such cruel losses. She understood that this was what she and her family had looked like, and that, a year later, they no longer did.

At Camp Ray of Hope, campers meet in groups of peers both Saturday and Sunday morning, each group led by two trained facilitators, and the groups are sometimes further arranged so that campers can be with others who have experienced a similar loss—a men's group, a widow's group, a group for grieving parents, a group for adolescent boys. Sometimes the groups find their own reason for being. The fall I attended, I was assigned to a group with two women whose sisters had both recently lost young sons. We were clearly together because we didn't fit in any of the other adult groups—the leftovers, really. But at our first meeting we realized we had much in common as grieving sisters and aunts, and labeled ourselves "the sisters' group."

Beyond the groups, the weekend offers a variety of

activities to grieving families, and, even as reluctant campers, the Kervins and I participated in many of these, as did my daughter. There are craft workshops for children and adults, massages, Reiki, and manicures, a No-Talent Show, a night walk without flashlights in the woods, canoeing and fishing, singing and s'mores around a campfire, a non-denominational worship service under the pines at the edge of the pond on Sunday morning. After lunch on Sunday there is a closing ceremony in a clearing in the woods, during which the families hang ornaments that they've created in honor of those they've lost on a small evergreen tree, and each family is given a monarch butterfly to release. Everyone stands in a circle, a community of the grieving.

Of their first year at camp, the Kervins mostly remember the experience of finally being with people who understood their grief—"new people, wanting to listen," as Adam describes them. He and Lori went into groups for pre-teens and teens, while Sandra and Ed met with other parents who had lost a child.

That weekend, the Kervins began to do what Ed describes as "the intense work that you need, but don't know you need." They met other parents who had survived sudden, unexpected tragedy. "A child is a gift from God," Ed tells me of his feelings then. "To lose a child is the worst thing that can happen to you. We were hoping desperately for a hand."

It was in the parent group that another father, who had lost his seventeen-year-old daughter, gave Ed his first words of hope. "Your pain will never go away," he told Ed, "but at some point in time it will become less severe."

Sandra sensed in the other campers their sincerity, their deep knowledge of pain, "a certain magic." She and Ed returned home, feeling they could go on. Something seemed possible that hadn't seemed possible before.

As the Kervins talk, I remember feeling the same sense of life opening a crack after Camp Ray of Hope. Our fast-paced American culture isn't kind to those who mourn. You have the funeral, flowers, a flurry of letters, and then—slam bang—you're expected to get on with your life as if nothing had changed. But this isn't how grief works. After my sister died, a friend, a minister, wrote me that he saw mourning as a long process of finding a place for the dead in our memories. Everyone at Camp Ray of Hope understands this—that grief takes work, attention, and time, but that sorrow can be eased by sharing your loss with others and by creating meaningful rituals.

I came to Camp Ray of Hope because of my sister's death, but I had actually brought with me a whole suitcase of losses. In addition to my mother four years earlier, cancer had claimed a close friend the previous winter, a month to the day before my sister's death. Then, in July, one of my oldest friends, an aid worker in Zimbabwe, was murdered in her home in Harare, possibly for political reasons. The world appeared intent, suddenly, on revealing itself as a place of random cruelty, piling up examples of violent and too-early deaths personal to me, just in case I'd missed the horrific accounts of wars and famines and accidents in the newspaper. I hadn't, but it's different, of course, when death creates great gaps in your own small world, and your family, once so comfortably ordinary, becomes one to whom tragedies happen.

The spring following my sister's death, the suggestion of a friend that I contact Dale Clark at Hospice proved a lifeline in keeping me from falling into deep despair. By the time I came to Camp Ray of Hope, I had, as Sandra and her children would a year later, a sympathetic bereavement counselor who listened week after week to my struggles, and I was receiving bereavement correspondence. But it was only in September, at Camp Ray of Hope, that I glimpsed what could easily appear a cliché, but which for so many participants proves deeply true—a sense that life still had meaning, a ray of hope. I understood that, while sorrow would never leave me, joy just might find its way into my heart again.

In the winter, two months after Jarod's death and eight months before the family would attend Camp Ray of Hope, Sandra unexpectedly discovered another lifeline. One afternoon in January, Lori begged to be taken shopping, so Sandra reluctantly drove her into Waterville, planning to wait in the car. Instead she found herself going into Mr. Paperback and asking one of the three clerks behind the counter if the store carried a book about a son's suicide that she'd heard about, *My Son, My Son*, by Iris Bolton. The clerk confided in Sandra that her own son had completed suicide in April, adding that she wanted to make a quilt out of his clothes someday.

Sandra remains amazed by the way this encounter might so easily not have happened—why this clerk, when she could have asked one of the other women? The thought of making a quilt captured her. She had learned quilting from her mother; quilting was something the two of them had done together all the time. Returning home, she told Ed she wanted to make a quilt out of Jarod's clothes. "I can't picture it," Ed said, but he gave the project his blessing.

That winter, she started the quilt. Some days, all she could do was just sit on the floor of Jarod's apartment and hold a piece of his clothing and cry. She moved the pieces around. She asked Lori and Adam and Ed to each design a square. Lori's square consisted of photographs of her with her older brother. Adam chose a note he'd written to Jarod the previous summer. Jarod had saved the note, which the family found in a drawer after his death.

Because the boys often played ball together—Jarod coached Adam's Little League team and helped Ed coach Adam's soccer team—Sandra took apart the baseball they'd often thrown and sewed the parts in a square with Adam's note. Ed chose a white shirt with matching suspenders and tie that he'd given Jarod, his first dress-up clothes. Sandra transferred Jarod's driver's license, fishing license, and the photographs, as well as the note from Adam, onto cloth and made them part of the quilt.

When she was finished, it measured six feet square and held hundreds of pieces of cloth from

Jarod's clothes—his jeans, his shirts, his under-shirts, his athletic socks, the logos from his T-shirts. At the center, she set his graduation picture from Lawrence High School, framing it with strips of cloth from the clothes he was wearing, his white T-shirt, his blue striped shirt, his blue jeans. In some of the patches, she arranged the pieces of clothing to suggest the way Jarod had worn them, the shirts open at the neck, the jeans coming down a bit in back, revealing the band of his boxers. "It was worse than a jigsaw puzzle," Sandra says. "Nothing was square." The quilt took five months and was the most intense piece of work she'd ever done. When it was completed, the Kervins had an open house and quilt signing on what would have been their son's 19th birthday, June 30. Jarod's friends and family friends and co-workers all came and wrote memories and messages of appreciation to Jarod on the quilt's back.

Two years after Jarod's death, in the fall of 2001, the Waterville Hospice offered a Survivors of Suicide group. (This was the group I co-facilitated, where Sandra and I first met.) Sandra decided to try a group again. She'd helped get her family as far as they'd come; now, she agreed reluctantly, she needed to work on her own grief. She was quiet in the group. Some sessions she still didn't feel like talking. But she stayed through the end, bringing to one of the last meetings a poem she'd come across that gave her consolation, "I'm Spending Christmas with Jesus this Year." The other group members, who had lost partners, a twin sister, and a father-in-law, found the poem so comforting that they requested copies.

Sandra and Ed took Hospice training to become volunteers in the fall of 2002; since then, they have gone to conferences for suicide prevention and for survivors and have led groups for bereaved parents both at the Hospice Community Center and at Camp Ray of Hope. They've become especially involved in helping those bereft by suicide, part of their mission to take away the shame and stigma of the act.

"We are willing," says Ed, "to go anywhere, anytime, to talk to anyone." They always bring the quilt. "We're known as the quilt people," Sandra tells me. They wrote about the quilt for the anthology, "Chicken Soup for the Grieving Soul," where the story was one of 69 chosen for publication out of 5,000 submissions. Sandra finds it telling that theirs is the only story in the book to mention suicide, despite the fact that 30,000 people take their own lives each year in the U.S., where suicide is the 11th most common cause of death.

Adam has also become very involved in Hospice. When I emailed Sandra to set up our first meeting, she wrote back asking if I could come on an evening when Adam could be there. "I hope you'll write about him," she said. "He's so much a part of our story." Last spring, Adam took Hospice volunteer training, and this September worked for a second time at Camp Ray of Hope with a group of adolescent boys, who were all about the same age he was when Jarod died. "People said to me, 'I'm here in case you fall.' Now it's time to reach my hand out," he explains of his decision. His first year working at the camp, he hadn't yet had Hospice training, and Sandra worried about that, but the director, Sue McConnell, who'd asked Adam to volunteer, assured her he'd be terrific, because he'd "lived it." "To have watched him struggle with the death and his own grief, we sit back in awe," Sandra tells me.

In their search to make sense of Jarod's death, "a reason for it all to happen," as Ed says, he and Sandra have found a direction for life after Jarod in reaching out to others and educating whoever will listen about suicide—how it can happen unexpectedly, how no family is exempt, how wrong it is that a suicide be stigmatized. They see themselves as continuing to honor Jarod's memory in their presentations, not letting him be forgotten. "There's another way to look at suicide," Sandra says of their message. While what they hope is to prevent a suicide, they also try to understand and respect those who choose to end their own lives. "It takes great courage to do what they do, not to turn away at the last second," Ed says to me. "It's got to be the most difficult decision to end a life, to struggle alone on your own battlefield. Think about what they have to muster inside to do that."

It's six weeks later and mid-November when I visit the Kervins again. Sandra already has the Christmas decorations up in the living room, Christmas figures on the mantel, a wreath ready to put on the door, a crèche, and the house looks and feels festive. When I arrive, Lori's daughter Ariel, now 20 months, is finishing her supper. Sandra and Ed and I sit in the living room, while Adam and Lori wander in and out, and Ariel runs around, bringing me her books. I had asked Sandra if I could see the quilt again, and so she takes it from where it's folded on the back of the couch and spreads it like a colorful rug across the carpet. It is, as it turns out, the first time Ariel has seen the quilt, and she sprawls across it, as if it's a huge picture book, pointing to various pieces and asking her favorite question, "Wassat?" She recognizes her mother, her "Grampy" and "Memere," her uncle Adam. Sandra points to pictures of Uncle Jarod. The grownups deter her when she wants to yank at the car keys dangling so enticingly from one of the squares, but otherwise the quilt is hers to explore.

The Kervins feel it's crucial that people not let a death, and particularly the manner of death, obscure the reality of the person who once lived—for them, a hard-working, generous, loving young man, a wonderful son and brother. "I wish you could have known my son," Ed tells me, and I assure him, though it's only a small bit of knowing, that because of the quilt and the memories and stories it evokes, I have a picture of their son—a thoughtful young man who loved sports and was admired by his parents and siblings. Although Adam and Jarod were six years apart, they played together often, especially outdoors, tossing a football in the backyard even in the snow. Jarod would tease Adam by calling him "Weiner" because he was then so small; for Adam's birthday, two months before his own death, Jarod gave him a card with "weiner" written all over the front, which Adam still treasures. It's also clear that right up until his death, Jarod led a packed life as a student and worker. He was a first-year student in a four-year program in business administration at Thomas College in Waterville, and hoped to own his own business someday. In addition to his studies, he worked 30–35 hours a week at the local grocery store and with Ed on Mondays at Service Merchandise in Augusta.

What happened to Jarod, what happened to them, says Sandra, could happen to anyone. The suicide mustn't be allowed to shadow the richness of all their son gave them. They now understand his death as a chemical imbalance in his brain, arising like a sudden mental illness. A priest who came to the house the day of the death suggested to the family as much, and for a long time, Sandra angrily dismissed his words. But she and Ed came to share the priest's theory after much reading and research, and after studying the letter they found in Jarod's apartment. Sometime during the night before he killed himself, Jarod wrote them a two-page letter on his computer, saying he loved them and explaining why he was taking his own life. He wrote the last paragraph by hand, which Sandra and Ed see as his way of leaving a personal text, "a last bit of love."

They found a box of tissues next to the computer, damp tissues in the wastebasket by the desk. "It must have been so strange and sad for him," says Ed.

On this visit, when Sandra spreads the quilt out on the living room floor, Lori, who was working in September when I visited, joins us. She has two new jobs now—at the Flower Cart and at the Dollar Tree, both in Augusta. (The Dollar Tree is a family theme—Adam is now assistant manager at the Dollar Tree in nearby Skowhegan.) Lori has not followed her younger brother and parents deeper into Hospice involvement. She went to Camp Ray of Hope with the family six years ago, when she was fifteen, and though she says it was a "pretty powerful weekend," hasn't returned. "It's good for first-time families," she tells me.

Lori is remarkably honest about the pain she felt and still feels about Jarod's death and its aftermath, the feelings of abandonment she had as a teenager, the anger and resentment she still carries about the loss of the family of her childhood. Her family, she tells me, totally changed. After Jarod's death, her parents weren't who they had been, "not even close." Living together again in one house is a rough patch that they are all hopeful about making their way through. Yet, despite the rawness she still feels, becoming a mother has given Lori insight into and empathy for her parents and what it must have been like for them. "Now that I have a kid," she says to me, "I can't imagine what it would be like to lose one."

"We couldn't be there for you, because we couldn't be there for ourselves," Ed says to Lori about the time after Jarod's death. As Lori talks, I think about how vulnerable we all are at fifteen—just beginning to establish an identity apart from our families, and yet still needing the comfort of home when the outside world appears hard and unforgiving. And yet for Lori, home had become a place of pain.

"Death can tear apart a family," she says to me, and while her presence in the room might seem to belie this truth, it's clear that for her the tearing apart is still the most important part of the family's story, and without this aspect, there would be something false in the telling. Sandra has patched together Jarod's life for the family in her extraordinary quilt, but this is, Lori indicates, her mother's quilt, not hers. It was her mother's idea that she do a square, she tells me, shrugging, when I ask about her contribution. She just found some photographs.

A quilt can cover things over, hiding as well as

comforting. While Ed and Sandra wish Lori would join them on their path through grief, they don't attempt to conceal her dissent. They understand that her experience has been different and, loving her as they do, they do not stop her from sharing it with me. Her pain is clear and poignant.

Lori asks me what I know about the ways people grieve from my work as a Hospice volunteer, and I stumble over my answer, talking about how individual grief is. It's only later that I remember a quotation to share with her, from a little book by Molly Fumia called *Safe Passage: Words to Help the Grieving Hold Fast and Let Go*:

"The season of our grief is our shutting down time. We prepare the cottage of our hearts for the winter, securing our windows to the world, stocking our cupboards with what will sustain us during the cold and dark. Carefully we rebuild our inner fire, and huddle in its warmth while the storms of winter pass, awaiting a spring that will come as surely as the steady passage of the days."

In this context, you might say that Ed and Sandra and Adam have glimpsed the spring, while Lori is still feeling the cold of winter, awaiting the spring as she bears witness to grief's persistence.

Or perhaps her daughter Ariel is the spring for all of them. It is moving to watch her, this child who has brought life back into a grieving house, as she acquaints herself with an uncle she will only know through stories. It strikes me that Ariel is Lori's gift to her family, as Adam's Hospice work is his. Ariel can never replace Jarod, but with this baby, Lori has brought her family another child to love. The first time I saw Sandra holding Ariel, at the Hospice Lights for Life gathering in December 2005, she was relaxed and happy, and her eyes carried a light that I'd never seen before in the four years I'd known her.

For the Kervins, Jarod is still so much a part of their family that when they had a family portrait done a few years ago, they knew they had to find a way to include him. Working with Elm City Photo in Waterville, they first had a color portrait done, then transposed Jarod's graduation photograph in black and white. In the foreground, Ed, Sandra, Lori, and Adam stand close together, smiling, while behind them Jarod seems to hover, much fainter, "an astral projection," as Lori says, as if he were keeping watch over them. The portrait sits on the mantel, and visitors to the house tend to look, then take a second look, says Sandra. A workman recently commented to her, "I think you have a ghost in your picture!" When she explained they'd lost their son, he was embarrassed, but Sandra assured him she was glad for a chance to talk about her son. "It's an honor and a privilege to continue to be Jarod's parents," Ed says.

At the end of the evening, I find myself telling the Kervins another road story, this one about my sister, who drove off into an ice storm on the night of January 14, 1999, pulled her car over on the shoulder near a Waterbury, Connecticut exit of I-84, and stepped or possibly slipped into the path of an 18-wheeler. The newspapers presented her death as a tragic accident, my sister a casualty of the ice storm. But the previous year she had been hospitalized twice for depression and a psychotic breakdown, and I'd been too worried about her for too long not to believe she'd found a way out of a life that—despite the love of her family and many friends—had become unbearable.

The Kervins are empathetic. Sandra says that she feels lucky that Jarod left a letter, so there is no ambiguity that his death was a suicide.

My sister was very devout, and she and I often talked about my own drifting away from the Christian beliefs in which we were raised. She was concerned about me, but tried to understand. Shortly after her death, a woman in the Episcopal church my father had attended for more than fifty years stopped him after a service and offered what she surely hoped were words of consolation. "God must have needed her more than she was needed on earth," the woman said. My father was appalled. More than her husband and her three sons? he wondered, perhaps asked out loud. He couldn't believe in or continue to worship a God whose plans included leaving a young family so bereft, and within a few months, he stopped going to church. He is still, he told me recently, unable to look at an album my sister made for him of his 75th birthday celebration, when our mother was still alive and all the children and grandchildren were there. "It makes me too sad," he said.

Unlike my father, the Kervins have not lost their faith in God and in divine providence—that everything on earth happens for a reason (though the reasons may not be fully understood, or only at a later time). When I tell them this story, they identify not with my father's turning away from God, but with the persistence of his pain. "It never goes away," Sandra agrees, "but we've learned to live without

Jarod." They try, she says, "to hold everything in a positive light."

This past summer, she had an encounter that also reminded her of the ways in which many people fail to understand the stubbornness of grief. She was at work at Inland Hospital, talking with a Vietnam vet with post-traumatic stress disorder who was struggling with insomnia. Sandra shared with him that she still has many sleepless nights herself. "Some nights are like that," she sympathized. Also in the room was someone who knew of Jarod's death. He looked at her in astonishment. "You're still bothered by that?" he asked.

Recently, my husband showed me a poem by the German poet Heinrich Heine. Heine evokes the mythical figure of Atlas, carrying the world on his shoulders, and describes him as one who must bear the unbearable, "das Unerträgliche tragen." I think of that image when I think of the Kervins, who like my father—and of course like me and the rest of our family—have struggled with questions of meaning after the loss of a beloved child. How does one bear such sorrow and remain open to life? How does one heal?

"Heal" is an Old English word meaning to be made whole. So perhaps one could say that Sandra, with her quilt composed of scraps of fabric from her son's clothes, has made something whole out of what had been broken, and that has been part of her healing.

And yet what has been made whole is not unchanged. Another domestic image, that of a broken teacup, evokes this truth in the literature of grief. The teacup may be mended, may even be used again, but the crack remains visible, marking its history. In this context, one might say that, through the grace of Hospice, the Kervins and other mourners have found a way of mending what death had broken in our lives.

For them, there is also great comfort in God's promise to re-unite them in the after-life with their son. This faith is so common among Hospice volunteers and clients that, soon after I started attending a Survivors of Suicide group, the November after my sister's death, I realized I was the only one who didn't assume I'd see her again. It took me three meetings to confess to being agnostic about an after-life. To my relief, everyone was sympathetic, but I also felt their sadness for me, as if, through some misunderstanding, I had to make my way through life truly unarmed and unconsoled. And yet, I don't feel that way, despite not knowing. I am confident that some time, as my minister friend suggested, I'll find a place for my sister in my memory that will bring me consolation. After all, what is memory if not a quilt?

Ed says that the memory of what they saw the morning of Jarod's death has faded for Adam, but not for him. Still, with that devastating image comes a more hopeful one. The image was given him by Dale Clark, now the Director of Hospice. A few years ago Dale, who lost her son Jonathan when he was seventeen, told Ed that she was picturing Jarod and her own son helping other young people make the crossing to "the other side."

As Ed tells me of this image, I imagine he is seeing Jarod as he appears in his graduation picture—a good-looking, dark-haired young man, smiling warmly, dressed in a blue striped shirt (left open at the neck) and jeans. He walks along another road, in a wooded landscape not unlike that of Camp Ray of Hope. Then he stops where a bridge crosses a stream, waiting for the too-young dead who are coming across to meet him.

"And Adam is here on this side helping other young people who are grieving." The image gives him great comfort. "I now have a son on each side, helping other young people," he tells me. "Both are very amazing souls."

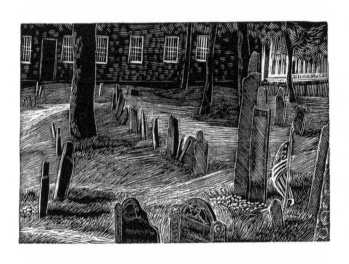

SWEET PEA
Bill Roorbach

I was sad. My mom had died in April, just a few months before, and that day driving over to Waterville (45 minutes straight east from Farmington) I was feeling it, living that phase of contemporary American mourning when the world around you says get on with it and you just can't: the sadness not only sticking but getting deeper, more layered, more profound, more awful, really, for the misconception that it was just going to suddenly lift. I couldn't concentrate enough to read, much less write, and anything I wrote seemed to have a mother looming.

And the day was chilly, bleak. I'd dressed up a little because Nancy Chamberlain was a hospice board member and that meant she was going to be really rich and put together, Ann Taylor blouse and subtle Coach bag and big black Mercedes, hair all poofed professionally.

And me in my Subaru wagon, 135,000 miles. And my little goofy beard and ponytail, not exactly what a grieving military mom wants to see. Oh, I was sad. Sad and self-conscious, too. Like, oh, I look like someone whose mom is dead. I'd had to stop in Norridgewock at a school—I think it was a school—and park in the lot to cry. That was what it had been like for several weeks, all this secret weeping. I'm falling apart months after Mom's funeral. Something's wrong with me, I know. Other people are done after a week or two. I had all the courage of a milkweed floater, an image I couldn't help, given all the seeds parachuting everywhere before the grim fall wind. The ridiculous idea that something about this hospice book project would be helpful to me somehow. I couldn't read, I couldn't write, I couldn't concentrate. And nothing about my mom's death was anything like I thought it was going to be, but this daily realization: we're toast, all of us.

All of us!

In a hundred years, maybe a hundred ten, every single last person alive today is going to be dead. Except maybe one or two who lived on yogurt and pine nuts and balanced on their heads (and they'll only last marginally longer): dead. That will be many more than six billion deaths, slaughter of unheralded proportions. Six billion! Where will our descendents find enough land for all the graves!

Such were my thoughts. I pulled into the little dirt parking lot at Hospice Volunteers of the Waterville Area headquarters and just sat. How scruffy everything is in our part of Maine! The building was plain, a house, really, one story. I left the car reluctantly, climbed up the pre-fab cement steps, and knocked. Nothing. After a few long minutes I tried the door, stepped in. No one. I shouted a hello. Still no one. I'd been there the week before, met the director, Dale, and had had a quick tour, knew where a bathroom was, used it with some little pleasure: it's been painted and decorated as a garden scene by a Hospice volunteer who does such things professionally, really cozy and beautiful. And I thought of the massage room, just a closet, really, where volunteers under stress could get rubbed and pummeled by another volunteer who was an accomplished masseuse. And the big board table built by yet another volunteer, filling a room remodeled and painted by volunteers. All these good people.

All doomed.

I shouted, "Hello?"

It's a place of trust. I wandered into the room Dale had said the kids' support groups were in. Kids! That was the worst of it. Kids who'd lost friends, siblings, parents. Everywhere art projects and the words of children: *sadness, hope, fury, forgiveness. Miss you. Love you.* The kids had made a quilt, too, sewn their small squares of sorrow into something warm and colorful and oddly hopeful, connected. I examined the flower pots Dale had explained: the kids smash them to represent shattered lives, then glue them together and paint them and decorate them to represent lives built anew, not quite the same but more beautiful for the ... trauma. I picked up one, then another and another, compelling, fragile things, terra cotta shards imperfectly reassembled into pots, most with angular new holes in them. And as I handled all that hurt, the scruffy feeling left me, then the despair, the free-floating anger. I blinked and found myself in the world.

Dale had heard me from back in her office, finished whichever of ten thousand tasks she was conquering, came bustling to see what was what. I was what was what, was what was what. She said the warmest hello, then just looked at me, pulled me in for a hug.

I had pictured Nancy Chamberlain wrongly, of

course. Her clothes were nice, but more J.C. Penney than Prada. Her hair was cut smartly, short and white, eyeglasses clean, eyes clear, direct. She looked like a head of nursing, which is exactly what she was, at St. Joseph Hospital over on North Street, no nonsense and generous all at once. She was sixty-four years old, unbowed, unbent, a little wary of me (or was I projecting—my mother always so wary?), warm nevertheless. We sat at opposite ends of a long, deep couch whose cushions had seen a lot of mourning. I noticed the tissue boxes everyplace. A lot had been confessed on this couch, a lot forgiven, a lot accepted.

Nancy crossed her legs, so I crossed mine. We leaned back away from one another. I asked questions, not exactly small talk, more like a police interview, I doing my best to be the good cop. I can report that she was calm under interrogation, dignified, a bit cool in the Yankee manner, though she warmed quickly as she spoke, and as I managed to relax.

"I live in Winslow," she said. "A new condo in Winslow. Across the Kennebec River from Waterville, our sister city. And they are competitive like sisters: who's best looking? Smartest?" Spoken by someone who knew from sisters.

What got her interested in hospice?

"Jay," she said. "Major Jay T. Aubin. My son."

Her son, I knew, was a helicopter pilot, a Marine. He'd been dead three and a half years, the first American casualty in the second Iraq War, the one marketed as "Iraqi Freedom." Which had since become the source of a great deal of mourning all around the globe.

But it wasn't quite time to talk about all that.

Dale had explained to me earlier that hospice is not only for the dying. It's for the living, too, support in a world that doesn't always understand grief.

Nancy said, "I'm a take-charge person. Always was. And I've always been the caretaker. I'm the oldest of fourteen children. I grew up in Skowhegan taking care of kids and babies from the time I can remember." Skowhegan is twelve miles upstream from Winslow/Waterville on the Kennebec. "And I've worked since I can remember, too, went off to nursing school at college age because that was what was available to me. And I worked as a nurse at St. Joseph for many years. After that I worked at Pollack Jewelers for six years."

Nancy was born a Willette, later married an Aubin, one who proved to be alcoholic. "Divorced him," she said with evident satisfaction. Later she married a man seventeen years her senior. And thus became a Chamberlain.

"I was fully retired. But one of the sisters at St. Joseph came to church—they knew they'd find me at church—came to church and found me. They asked me to come back as director of nursing. And in truth I'm happy to be back. It's more of a calling, more of a duty, more spiritually satisfying. The jewelry store was fun and social but of course very material, materialistic. I was working there when...."

Captain Jay T. Aubin died March 21, 2003 (his promotion to major was posthumous). Nancy didn't quite say the words, but it was clear enough what she meant.

"We weren't supposed to know where he was, but we did, because Colonel Oliver North was embedded not only in his unit but in his tent. You remember Oliver North. Well, this was his new role as Fox reporter. I got a phone call at the Pollack, from a co-worker. She said, oh, 'A helicopter has gone down.' And I just thought, Well, there are thousands of helicopters in Iraq right now. No reason to think... And I finished up there at work and went home. Put on Fox News. Hoping for a glimpse of Jay. We'd been watching Fox all along, hoping for glimpses. He'd said to us, 'Who knows? Maybe Ollie North will make me famous!' *Pathetic*!"

She half smiled, shaking her head, but only half, or maybe a quarter. Once, perhaps, the whole thing had seemed funny.

"He'd told me over and over never to worry about

the telephone, that I'd never hear from the Marines by telephone. That if anything happened, the Marines would come to the door to tell me. Now, remember, I'm a take-charge kind of person, someone who likes to take care of people. And my daughter-in-law calls from Arizona, Jay's wife, Rhonda, from the base in Arizona, and she says 'Do you have a support person there?'

I mean, he was a flight instructor safely based in Arizona, is how I'd seen it, and I'd been naïve enough to think he'd never have to go to war, that they'd need him there in Arizona, to teach others how to fly.

"I told her, 'I'm going to stay up all night and watch television. And if I hear anything at all, I'll call you.'

"And then, no more than 45 minutes later, I suddenly think, Rhonda knows something. So I called her back…. And a Marine Corps captain answers the phone. Captain Dillon—they send a person of equal rank. I didn't want to talk to him. I said put Rhonda on. And I said, 'Rhonda, it's not *Jay*?'

"And she said, 'They think so.'

"So I said, 'Put Captain Dillon back on.' And he got on and I said, 'I'm his mother. You just tell me. Was he killed?'"

"And Captain Dillon said, 'Yes Ma'am.'

"This was maybe 10:30 at night."

I eyed the tissue box, size large, didn't see how I could go for one just at that moment. If Jay could be tough, if Colonel Dillon could be tough, if Rhonda could be tough, I could be tough, too. What difference if my eyes leaked a little?

Nancy's face went softer, her gaze finding the darkening window, her thoughts flying far from the room, far from our interview, far from me and whatever I might be feeling, rightly so. She went on: "I don't remember what I said. Something very calm. And I hung up. Then I just started screaming. Really screaming, something I've never done. Screaming for my husband. He's a really good man. But he didn't know how to provide me with support. And you know, Jay was not only not his *son*, Jay was already out of the house and on his own by the time Chamberlain and I got together. And my husband just didn't have the faintest idea of what to say or do. And I am *screaming*. Finally, I called my sister Terry.

"She didn't recognize my voice! She said, 'Who is this?'

"And I'm saying, 'It's *Jay*, It's *Jay*!

"And she's thinking, Jay who? And then she gets it.

"Terry called the other sibs, we all live near, still, and within half an hour all twelve of us were there, including my 81-year-old mom. By eleven p.m. they're all there. I mean. And I'd called my priest—Father Paul Plante from Saint John the Baptist Catholic Church there in Winslow—and he was at my house in minutes and stayed with me for the half hour before they all arrived. Later Terry said she was thinking, What if I dreamed all this? Hoping she dreamed it all, so it wouldn't be true: What if I dreamed all this and I've gotten all these people here for no reason? The dream idea, it's a way to push the shock back. What if I dreamed it? Twelve people heading for Winslow and it was all a dream!

"If only.

"I had a nice den, and people had gathered in there watching Fox News, and I just went in and said, 'Turn off the TV!' Half my siblings wanted to watch. Half didn't. Even at the time, even in the emotion of the time I observed that. But I wanted it off. So they turned it off. Then I went in the kitchen for a minute. When I returned, the TV was back on, and my *seat* was taken. So my sister put a big sign on the TV:

KEEP TV OFF!

"The next morning I went to mass at seven. Father

Plante asks me, Do you want me to remember him to the congregation?

"And I said, 'Not till the Marines come.'

"I mean, I was still holding out hope, still in denial. And of course, the Marines did come; they came to the house while I was at mass. Later they came back. And later still I learned that they'd discussed whether to come in the middle of the night, the night before. The Marine in charge, a Major Ross, had heard about the helicopter accident, and that someone dead was from Maine. And there were two others from Maine that night. He told me he thought, How will we handle three of them? Had to ask *me* where Jay's dad was. Texas, but that's another story.

"I get home from church and everyone says, 'The Marines have been here, they'll be back.'

"They wouldn't stay. They had a chaplain with them and a driver, also Major Ross. I remember thinking, a *major*!

"I kept thinking how proud I was that Jay had made major, but at the same time how he wasn't, in fact, going to get to be a major.

"I had a couple of almost panic episodes: My God, they're going to blame Jay for the helicopter crash!

"My brother, Peter Willette, said, 'This is going to

be big, guys, we'd better start planning. He's first in the nation. We've got to think. For example: who's going to handle the interviews and stuff?'

"And I said, '*I* want to do the interviews. I want them to know what they do coming into our living rooms every night with these pictures from the war. *Every night.* Let them know what I *feel*.'

"And then out of the blue, *Tom Brokaw* called late Friday afternoon. This was a live feed and he was sitting with several generals. He said he was calling to give condolences. And at the very end of the interview I said, 'May I tell you something?' And he said to go ahead. So I said, 'All this shock and awe is wonderful, but you've got to remember that you've got mothers, fathers, families watching television looking for their children, for their relatives over there, watching this explosion and that crash and the other plume of smoke. But Tom, you can't imagine sitting there thinking, *Is that my son?*'

"Tom Brokaw, he broke down on television. Sitting with the generals. Later he called back, just himself, off the air. He said, 'Could I stay in touch?' And the network attached our earlier conversation to a video tape. NBC claims it did a lot of good in the way they reported things afterward. When Tom retired he dedicated his book to Jay and me, which was more credit than I deserved. He told me I'd done as great a service as Jay had. But I know that's not true. I was just a mother thinking about all those other mothers and fathers." Nancy gave me a long look, struggling with pride, it looked like to me, a truly modest person overtaken with the fact of her own pride, her gaze steady, oblique, her eyes expecting judgment, unafraid of judgment, vulnerable, too, these impossible combinations grief piles upon us.

"You're a good person," I said.

She looked doubtful, but went on: "I went to Tom's book party. And for a whole year NBC News would call to get my opinion on events in the war. When Hussein was captured, for example. What I thought was, Thank God Jay didn't go for nothing!

"But the way the war has gone! The atrocities charged to Marines. Bill, I'm glad Jay doesn't know about all of that. When we got into the war, Jay would say, oh, 'We Marines know more than you do. This is for the good of the Iraqi people.' Bill, he really believed that, really thought he was doing good.

"When we hit 2000 deaths, I was called again."

Long silence. I see the cracked pots, the letters to loved ones in crayon. The room is growing dim with dusk.

Nancy said as much to the room as to me, "I'm

angry. I don't know exactly why." Another long pause. She doesn't look angry. What she looks is tired. She looks soulful. She looks hungry. She looks mortal. I think of my mother, ineluctably, think of her upon the mention of anger. She'd grouse at her caregivers, excoriate my poor dad. And that anger in some way has been passed on to me. I can't contain it, but try, keep pushing down on the manhole cover as hard as I can, all day. But in the dark the anger heaves up, steam spouting from cracks in the cast-iron, fire spitting from the vents: odd pronouncements, careless driving, strange fears.

Nancy said, "This past weekend the "Young Marines" were out, these *little* kids doing fundraisers. I'm sorry, but I *wouldn't talk to them*. I thought, *Go be a kid, grow up first, then decide.*"

Later, nearer the end of 2006, I went to see Nancy in her new home, a smart condo on former pasture land in Winslow, a little north of town. There are more condos going in, and small trees planted and lights on in maybe half the homes, a sense of rebirth, hopeful growth, a lot of pipe and lumber lying around and cable groping up out of the ground for future streetlights. A week before I'd been in my own hometown down in Connecticut, and seen my parents' house, the house I'd grown up in, the house my mother had died in, the house my dad had just sold, already pasted with big signs:

NOTICE OF INTENT TO DEMOLISH

Later, in January, I'd stop by again and find the old homestead *gone,* a steam shovel—are they still called steam shovels?—a steam shovel digging a new foundation where the old place had been. Beloved huge oak trees gone. Gardens gone. Garage gone. Everything gone.

Erasure.

But these condos—clean and fresh and well-made. Nancy has thoroughly moved in—you wouldn't guess it's only been three months. She answers the door in a cute Christmas sweater, shakes my hand with an air of command, a welcoming practical confidence, not quite a smile, eyeglasses polished, hands washed. There are signs of a dog—a plastic porkchop, a hanging leash—but no dog to be seen. There are also signs of a husband—coat, hat, a minor note of something male in the air. But no husband to be seen. First thing I notice as I cross the threshold is a little porcelain dish inscribed, "We Love You."

Nancy and I repair a few paces to her office, a dining room really, or maybe a TV nook, set up with her computer and a couple of comfy chairs, also an antique baby carriage with an antique porcelain doll lying in it, the kind my daughter calls a "look-at" doll. "My mother gave me that after Jay died," Nancy said. And we hold an expressive silence. After a while she sees I'm looking at the wall behind her, where I've spotted a wooden figure of a helicopter, also a case full of medals. She says, "I didn't want to have a shrine. Just a few tasteful things."

And the display is tasteful, a kind of short introduction to the lost man. I get up for a close look. A beautiful maple case (made by one of Jay's friends) contains his many military awards. At the top is the Purple Heart, received for that most grievous wound, his death. And then two rows of less exalted medals, many received during earlier tours of duty in Desert Storm/Desert Shield: Navy Commendation Medal with Gold Star and "V" for Valor in Combat; Navy Achievement Medal; Good Conduct Medal; National Defense Service Medal; Armed Forces Expeditionary Medal; Southwest Asia Service Medal; Global War on Terrorism Expeditionary Medal; Humanitarian Service

Medal; Saudi Arabian Defense Medal; Kuwait Liberation Medal.

And two rows of ribbons.

Also a brass plaque:

> MAJOR JAY T. AUBIN
> "SWEET PEA"
> AN AMERICAN HERO
> "DOING WHAT HE LOVED"
> SO THAT OTHERS MAY BE FREE
> SEMPER FIDELIS

Nancy sighs. "His call signal was Sweet Pea, and Sweet Pea was what they all called him. Imagine, in that tough culture, someone man enough to be called Sweet Pea!"

And there's a wood-burning from a fellow Marine—Jay's likeness, trans-copied from a photograph. And the last little thing Nancy has chosen to display (from a nearly endless supply of possibilities): a photo, taken in East Timor by a flying colleague, Jay piloting his helicopter in front of a cliff-top cathedral, nearly in the arms of a huge statue of Jesus raising his hands to the sky.

A Healing Touch

Nancy says, "I've got four legal-size letter bins, these huge plastic letter bins, full of memorabilia. Cards, articles from papers. Video of the CNN story, endless other stuff. I hardly know what to do with it all. Letters from just about everyone you can think of. Senator Snowe, Senator Collins, Senators not even from Maine, Representative Michaud, Representative Allen, Governor Baldacci, General Mike Hagee, Commandant of the Marine Corps."

She's thought of something. She leaves me on my own, looking at the ribbons. I can hear her rummaging in a back room. Soon she reappears with a large scrapbook. "One of my sisters made this for me." It's prodigious: articles from all the Maine papers, the Boston papers, from *Newsweek*, the same few recurring photos. Jay made a tough-looking Marine, it's true, but there's something very sweet indeed shining through, something human and warm and wonderful, no matter how formal the pose.

And he made a handsome civilian dad, as evidenced by another photo, a shot of him sitting on a California beach with his wife, Rhonda, daughter Alicia (who was 10 when he died), son Nathan (who was 7). I flipped the pages, came to photos of the funeral service in San Diego, where Rhonda and he had hoped to live upon his return, her home town, one of his many bases, Rhonda crying, hugging Alicia, erect Nathan a few steps away in each picture, standing alone, hugging to his chest an American flag properly folded.

The newspaper columns saved in the scrapbook made note of Nancy's cautionary words to Brokaw, but the message of their outraged punditry is unclear: should the TV news people merely be more careful about what they show, or should they be more careful about what they promote, both consciously and unconsciously? There's a note of outrage, but the target of the outrage isn't clearly defined.

From one of his young cousins, Adrianna Willette, felt-tip pen:

> I really never knew him but I still loved him.
> I nearly cried when I heard he was gone. I felt
> awfel. My tears flowed down the sides of my
> cheeks. I'm sorry Aunt Nancy!

From Major John Graham, who was with him in Kuwait, a more than just obligatory note to the mother of a fallen comrade:

> I will always fondly remember that warm,

but somewhat goofy smile and funny sense of humor. He was a true patriot and respected by all.

From Dennis Willette, one of Nancy's brothers, Jay's uncle: "No man is perfect but in our human eyes, Jay had a real good start."

Not in the scrapbook, but framed and hung on the wall in a back bedroom, a piece of paper signed in a big hand by the Commander in Chief:

The United States of America honors the memory of Jay Thomas Aubin.
This Certificate is awarded by a grateful nation in recognition of devoted and selfless consecration to the service of our country in the Armed Forces of the United States
George W. Bush

"Sad. This hole in my life, it'll never be filled. He was my oldest son. He was my best friend in the world. I have three sons. Jay was the achiever. He—we— couldn't afford college, but the Marines paid for that. He went to school, came back an officer. My first husband was an alcoholic, as I've told you. Jay always filled a certain role for me. He was my first baby."

Sweet Pea was born August 8, 1966, in Skowhegan. He attended the Skowhegan Area High School, where he was very popular among teachers and students alike. "Always a smile on his face," according to Dennis Hart, who was his wrestling coach. "He was determined to be the best that could be at anything he tried." He made Student of the Year his senior year, no mean achievement.

He enlisted in the Marine Corps in March 1984.

In her den, Nancy said, "Captain Dillon was such a help. He called, he visited. He said I could see Jay's remains if I wanted. I knew I had to see Jay, that I wouldn't believe he was dead until I saw him. But in the end I just couldn't. I regret it now. He's buried in San Diego. And the hearse. I understand now why people throw themselves on coffins. But I didn't. I did not. I didn't want to touch the flag: always the good girl. I'm a little angry at myself for that."

Immediately after the funeral in San Diego there was a memorial service at the Marine Corps Air Station Chapel in Yuma, Arizona, where he'd last been stationed, where Rhonda and the kids lived. The bulletin for that day's service shows a recent picture of their fallen comrade, a clean-cut soldier standing at ease unsmiling, but with an unmistakable cheer about him—once again!—a kind of grin welling up because of the presence of the photographer (whose place we take as we look), neatly pressed camo fatigues, five o'-clock shadow on his cheeks and chin, blue eyes, heavy eyebrows, wings over his pocket, the kindliest face I've ever seen in uniform.

The bulletin carried a military obituary, as well, missing a comma or two, but heartfelt, and full of information, which I'll reproduce in full for its window on what a certain culture finds important, skim if you wish:

Major Jay Aubin enlisted in the Marine Corps in March 1984 and began Recruit Training at Marine Corps Recruit Depot Parris Island, South Carolina in Feb 1985. After graduation from Recruit Training, he was trained as an Aircraft Mechanic on the A-6/AE-6 aircraft and served with Marine Attack Squadron (All Weather) (VMA(AW)) 242 at Marine Corps Air Station El Toro, California until his transfer to the Marine Corps Reserve in 1989. Major Aubin was called back to active duty during Desert Storm and served until May 1991. While attending the University of Southern Maine, he was enrolled in the Platoon Leaders Class. He graduated with a

Bachelors Degree in Industrial Technology.

In December 1993 Major Aubin was commissioned a Second Lieutenant in the United States Marine Corps. Upon his commission he attended The Basic School from August 1994 to February 1995. Upon completion of the Basic School, he transferred to NAS Pensacola, where he underwent Naval flight training. On 13 December 1996, Major Aubin completed flight training and earned his wings as a Naval Aviator. He was subsequently transferred to Marine Helicopter Training Squadron 204 (HMT-204) at Marine Corps Air Station New River, NC for follow-on training as a CH-46 Sea Knight helicopter pilot.

Major Aubin's Fleet Marine Force time was spent with Marine Medium Helicopter Squadron 265 (HMM-265) in Okinawa, Japan from September 1997 to May 2002. During his time with HMM-265, Major Aubin attended the Weapons and Tactics Instructor Course at Marine Aviation Weapons and Tactics Squadron One, graduating in April 2000 only to return in July 2002 to serve as a CH-46 Weapons and Tactics Instructor.

With the deployment of Marine forces to

Kuwait for participation in operation Enduring Freedom (later named Iraqi Freedom), Major Aubin was requested by Marine Aircraft Group 39 (MAG-39) to provide planning and execution expertise and served with Marine Medium Lift Helicopter Squadron (HMM-268) during hostilities.

Nancy remembers the service: "The Marine Corps did a tremendous job. We heard so many things about Jay. Huge crowd, over six hundred, mostly women, wives of Marines—the men of course were gone. That's where we learned they called him Captain Sweet Pea. He was *Sweet Pea*! He did so many things and never told us. One story was about the last Marine Corps ball. Jay checked out a vehicle from the motor pool just so his people wouldn't be driving home drunk. I mean, Jay never drank—never—his father and all. And so he brought Rhonda home and then went back to the ball and drove those drunk Marines home in shifts. That was Jay. My Sweet Pea."

There's another scrapbook, one I didn't see, filled with documents and articles pertaining to the investigation of the helicopter crash. She repeated that she did not want to see Jay blamed for that crash, and didn't want to see any investigation go that way.

And it shouldn't, of course. First point of evidence, the Sea Knight helicopter. This is the craft Jay piloted, one of 239 in the Marine fleet at the time he died, all being phased out for replacement in September 2004 (though as I write in February 2007, the news comes that a Sea Knight has crashed in Baghdad killing all seven aboard: mechanical failure). The last new Sea Knight was built in 1974, the year the Vietnam war ended so precipitously. In the field, these large machines are called frogs, for their amphibian faces. The average age of the aircraft was 34 years when Jay went down, March 21, 2003. His own age was 36.

Over the not-shrine Nancy's got her own message hung, a quote from a familiar hymn: "Let there be peace on earth, and let it begin with me."

Back on the couch at Hospice Volunteers headquarters. It's getting dark, but Nancy makes no move to turn the lights on, and I don't either. We're the only ones in the place. A light's on in the kitchen, makes a glow. And there's a warm current running between us. I've sidetracked our talk, told Nancy a little about my own grieving, and it turns out she's just very good at listening, seems to have no need to step in with advice, no need to put it all into words. She just nods and waits, watches, listens. I feel seen. I feel heard.

You learn something every day: hospice is not only for the dying.

When it's her turn again, she seems almost reluctant to go on, but does: "In the middle of all this insanity—all this Brokaw and Senator Snowe and shock and family and avalanches of mail—I get a phone call, this soft-voiced person: Dale Clark. She wanted me to know about Hospice Volunteers. She said she knew it was way too soon, but just wanted to know if I'd like to get their mailings. They send notes out at three months after a death and six and twelve and fifteen, I think. Not the kind of thing I thought I would ever do, but I joined a six-week group. And I'd never walked into a place where I felt so warm, so accepted for being what I was. My group was three mothers who had lost sons, and one who'd lost two sisters. I stayed away from my feelings those six weeks. I didn't want to be part of that sorority. I only had to hear and see their pain—that helped me realize I'm not the only one, that my loss was no greater than theirs.

"But mine *was* different. Jay had been away for five years. That absence still interferes with proper grieving, I think.

"Our facilitator had had her losses too. All facilitators have had losses. So, they can relate. What the group is, is it's mutual support, guidance through the stages of grieving; it's validation for all those dark feelings, for my sense of going insane; it's contacts. You're with people who know what you've been through. That was the only group I joined, because of the way I am: I need to take care of other people, not be taken care of."

Long pause.

"Of course, taking charge is a way of grieving, too."

Nancy lets a self-deprecating, wry smile steal over her face. She's the head nurse again. But now I see the compassion, and really *boundless* heart; there is eternity there, right there in Nancy's smile. She says, "A year after one's own loss, one can volunteer. I took the course—thirty hours—jumped in with both feet. The following April. And this helped me cope. I worked in the office two days, got interested in grieving children. In June, I did the Hope's Place training, thirty more hours." Hope's Place is a program of Hospice Volunteers that helps grieving children. "I walked in to the second class, having missed the first for some reason. Here I am! The stranger!

"That training program began to crack the surface.

I was rather surprised, almost like an onlooker, as my own denial began to crumble."

She gave a short cough, frowned briefly with her thoughts, said, "And I always know the day's going to come when I'll feel that pain again. But I've got support. That original group of Hope's Place volunteers has given me so much. We've become so close. We're like sisters. I probably dealt with more of my grief here than anywhere.

"I'm currently a facilitator for a grieving children group. It's the fourth group I've done. These are ten-to-twelve week sessions. We meet right here. Hope's Place is a concept, but this is its home, the actual place." Cracked and painted flower pots, letters to lost loved ones, art projects all over the walls, the embodiment of hope.

"The parents are in one room, the boardroom over there, the one with the big table. The children are in here. And the parents are also grieving, of course, scared they're not doing the right thing. That's where I want to be, with the parents." Another wry smile. "Putting me in with the little kids, that would be a joke. I'm not the warm, fuzzy, mother type. No. Not growing up with thirteen babies to take care of. Give me the adults. Parents, grandparents in their mid-fifties who suddenly find themselves raising a toddler, aunts and uncles, those are the people I'm here to help."

In the dusk of the living room of Hospice Volunteers Headquarters, Nancy pauses. Her face is practically a movie of all the sad people she's seen and helped, and I watch. At length, she says: "There are nineteen children in the current session. And, oh! One little boy—four years old—he walked in here, and he planted his feet, and he said, 'My Daddy's dead and I'm mad at God!'"

Something funny in that, and we laugh, but ruefully.

"Now I'm on the board of Hospice Volunteers. They asked. I'm an organized person, with something to offer. I like the policy and planning committee, so I'm on that, too."

It's really getting dark. We sit in our thoughts once more, not long. That little boy mad at God? That's me. And any little boy, of course, any little boy at all, including that little four-year-old—for Nancy on some level he's got to be Jay. Major Jay T. Aubin, United States Marines.

Before long, Nancy speaks. It's a near whisper but I can hear her just fine in the quiet of the room, in the quiet of the evening: "The Marines were wonderful. But good as those services were out west, Yuma,

San Diego, I knew I had to bring it to closure here in Maine. This was Jay's home. I talked to Father Plante—and he got the whole church involved. They went to so much trouble. He got the Marines involved, the Winslow police. Another six hundred people! And I got a call from the fire department: 'We have an enormous American flag, may we fly it in front of the church?'

"Of course!

"The public part was okay. A full Marine service. What touched me most was that, as we drove into town to the church, all the flags they use for Fourth of July were lined along the streets all the way. All four choirs were there at St. John's. Everybody wanted to be there. There were eighty or a hundred of us just from the family! Mother went, and the older grandchildren.

"I know I told you I hadn't seen him in the five years before he died, but he did come home that July—just a four-day visit. He said, 'Mom, there's a question that I might be able to fly the president, so the FBI will be calling on you for a background check. Just be warned! I'm not in trouble or anything!' And then he went back to his high school, visited all over town, all the friends of his youth, all his cousins, grade school teachers, high school teachers, all of it in four days, all high-speed, very thorough. I think there was some kind of premonition—something deep inside, something driving him. Listen:

"At the hospital I do some bereavement work, too. I was out visiting the family of an older gentlemen, and suddenly realized he was the one who'd delivered Jay's last letter, our postman. The letter, oh, it was written over there. He said, 'If anything happens to me, just please stay in touch with Rhonda and Nathan and Alicia. I want them to know my Maine family.'"

And just for his mom:

I want to thank you for everything over the years. You always tried your best to put us first at your expense. I wish it had worked out that I was closer home to your grandkids. Hopefully, I will be home soon now that we are getting started.

"And this elderly man whose family I was visiting as a grief counselor, that same man was outside my door as I came out on the way to Jay's service. That postman was standing there, just about to knock. I nearly bowled him over. He said, 'We thought you might want to have this today.' And handed me what turned out to be Jay's last letter. I read it on the spot. Oh! Jay shared things he'd never shared. Things I'm not going to tell you. Then at church, before the service, I showed the letter to Father Paul. I gave him a portion to read at the service, a part in which Jay thanked his friends. The rest was too private. Just that the last words were, 'Thanks, Mom.'

"Later on I went to the PO to thank them, thank the postmaster, a woman. I wanted her to know, wanted all of them to know how good it was to have that letter. She said, 'Oh, you know, we stood around trying to decide whether to deliver it at that time or not. Some were for it, some against. But I said, "I'm a mother! She needs that letter!"'

"And the post office knew me, of course. I'd gotten something like 2000 cards and letters from all over the country, all over the world. From Kenya, Paris, Britain. People were praying for Jay and for us all over the world!"

The living room at Hospice Volunteers headquarters had gone nearly dark, just the glow from the kitchen, cold light from the street. Outside, cars and trucks stopped and started in waves for the traffic light on the corner, people going home from work, people heading out to evening shifts, hither and yon, engines racing.

I had one more question, asking, really, for my own sake: "Nancy, are you like that four-year-old boy? Are you mad at God?"

She answered without hesitation. This was something she'd thought about. "I've never been able to be mad at God. I'm just too good a girl. He took Jay, and Jay is with my Dad now, in a better place."

But she'd spoken of anger, so I said, "Are you mad at George W. Bush?"

Again, the quick answer: "I wasn't at first. I actually felt badly for him. Now, though, I'm totally confused. I don't want to think this war is about oil, or politics. I know one thing, though: whatever else was going on, Jay was doing it for the right reasons. He was doing it to help people. And he really, really believed in it. He believed it so much that it doesn't matter what the politics are. And he did help people. He helped people wherever he went. He was there to help, and I believe he did."

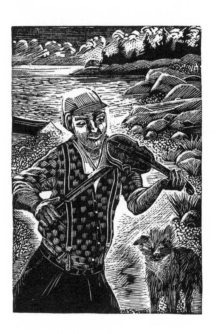

BLUE ANGELS, BLUE ANGELS

Monica Wood

When I ask Ellen Bowman to sing, she begins with a story.

Imagine a tiny girl in Ellen's office. Imagine her somber eyes, her wrinkled shirt, her precisely tied shoes. Imagine her father swaddled on his deathbed. "Blue angels flew in my daddy's room," this child tells Ellen. "Blue angels from the sky." Together, they remake the vision into a song, which, long after the father's death, Ellen sings to me:

> *Blue angels, blue angels, flying in my daddy's room*
> *I saw them, helping my daddy, blue angels in my daddy's room.*

Ellen's voice, a creamy alto, lifts above a breeze

that buffets a glowing patch of beach on a warm October day. We're seated on a trunk of driftwood that rests among a scattering of tide-burnished rocks. Her voice carries over the rocks, the waterfoam, the damp sands. I take up a harmony, and for a few moments time stops, as it will for music. Her song strikes me as an act of generosity—both toward that little girl at the time of her father's death, and toward me, now, on this scrap of beach where I'm looking for a way to write about dying. Ellen's voice sounds like an open door.

After we finish talking and walk the half block to her parents' house where she's visiting for the weekend, Ellen demonstrates one of her musical tools. She enlists her husband, Phil, a cellist who, at the moment, is helping Ellen's mother, Ruth, sort through tag-sale items in the garage. "Phil," Ellen says. "Can we—?" They lock eyes. He begins to vocalize—it's not exactly singing, but I can tell he's a tenor with the kind of clear-water voice made for choral music. Ellen adds a pleasing counterpoint and the garage fills with sound. In a setting of jumbled plant pots and rejected chairs, music happens. This is a "tone piece," kept aloft by tonal and nearly invisible physical cues that keep the vocalists from crashing into each other. They sing for about two minutes as Ruth and I listen. They form words that aren't words, just oohs and aahs and yays and yahs, and when they finish, I imagine how I would feel if I were dying. Anointed. Safe. Embraced by sound.

Before I leave, Ruth invites me into the house. She is tall and big-boned, with the posture of a redwood. An artist herself, connected and vibrant, she's wearing a wheat-colored sweater and longish skirt with a flashy belt cinched just below the waist. She could be one of those L. L. Bean catalog models except for her age, which turns out, astonishingly, to be ninety. In her dining room hang ancestral portraits of squat, expressionless matrons with big, round heads, their hairdos topped by the same flimsy headgear that looks like a starched hanky. They don't seem quite up to the task of begetting relatives, least of all a treelike woman who lives near a southern Maine beach, yet here are Ruth, and Ellen, too, a lineage of living, breathing people. The hanky-wearers have all died, but on the day they were painted they might have just chased a crow from the herb garden or made tea for the bishop. What happened at their bedsides, in the end? They look so unsuspecting, so sure of their continuing days.

I am writing this piece because of a promise. Someone I like and respect gave me a list of people connected to hospice and asked me to profile one of them. After dragging my heels for two solid weeks I recognized how premature was my consent. I didn't want to write about dying. Nobody I love died well.

The first person I contacted was Karen, a volunteer counselor for grieving children. Her own mother died when Karen was ten, and from her visceral retelling I can see how those feelings of shock and loss still linger. As we talk, my inner clock winds back more than thirty years, to 1974, where it turns into a real clock—that loud ticker in my family's kitchen in Mexico, Maine. My mother is dying. I've just arrived home from college for the Thanksgiving weekend. She's turned the color of ochre—my mother who always had such soft and peachy skin—and after saying hello to me, the last one home, she begins her goodbye, slipping beneath a coma from which she speaks only in rhythmic, sonorous breaths, so deep they appear to be hauling up all the water from the well of her life—not a long one—and we have only to wait for that well to empty. On the Sunday after Thanksgiving, at eight o'clock at night, it does.

My sisters and I didn't know the word "hospice." We knew nothing about dying well. During the four years of our mother's ordeal—she'd been paralyzed by a stroke after her first operation—we never once uttered the word "cancer" in her presence. We did not sing at her bedside. We were musical girls, trained in our church choir. And yet we did not think to sing.

Because Karen's and my stories intersect too tenderly, I skip down the list to Chuck, a handy, affable fellow who builds coffins disguised as shelving units. Imagine those planks being reassembled on a moment's notice, whip bang, to reveal their not-so-hidden purpose. Life is about evading death, but Chuck will have none of that. We speak by phone, and I picture him as a lumberjack in a plaid jacket. In reality he's a librarian, and I decide he'll make a dandy, smooth-sailing subject for an essay.

Then I meet Ellen, a freelance music therapist with that maple-syrup voice and those gold-brown eyes and that noteworthy mother. If a former choir girl has to write about death, she might as well buddy up with someone who can carry a tune. We meet. We sing. We begin.

When Ellen visits a hospice client for the first time, she peeks into closets and pokes behind doors: is there a banjo? an abandoned mandolin? a hymnal? What's that under the tarp? Good lord, a griefstricken grand piano, greasy with disuse. Who played it? In the home of an ancient, mute, dying woman named

Barbara Ann, Ellen removes the tarp, rummages inside the piano bench, unearths stacks of sheet music and plunders them for inspiration. Two hospice nurses, taking great pains, bundle Barbara Ann into a chair and wheel her pianoside. For Barbara Ann the woman, Ellen plays "Barbara Ann" the song. Eight bars in, Barbara Ann the woman, weak of limb and translucently white, hauls up one of her bloodless bird legs and smacks one slippered foot down on the bench, as if to say, "Dig it, honey!" Bingo. Ellen laughs. Her days vibrate with moments like this.

For Robert, a dentist transplanted from Brooklyn, Ellen commandeers another piano and wings through the score of *West Side Story*.

For Linda, a child of the sixties who wants the sound of California, Ellen turns up her old Joni Mitchell albums and a CD of shushing waves.

For Bill, an old soldier at the veterans' home, Ellen reproduces "The Cow Cow Boogie."

For Annie, an aged ornithologist, Ellen brings recordings of birds: birds accompanied by cellos, birds accompanied by violins, birds accompanied by nothing but the shivering trees from which they sing.

If Ellen had peered into my family's doorway in

1974, she would have spotted my guitar. I played with my friend Denise, for money—two folkies in peasant dresses singing Simon and Garfunkel—but our mothers preferred the cornball tunes we'd sung at the Grange hall back in our uncool early adolescence. "The Cruel War Is Raging," "Down in the Valley," "Where Have All the Flowers Gone," "Red River Valley"—no war or valley escaped our three-chord treatment. My sisters sang, too. At St. Theresa's Parish we did four-part Tantum Ergos and O Sanctissimas, possibly the last congregation in the country to succumb to the bland, committee-written, English-language Catholic hymns of the seventies. And, like all families, we had what Ellen calls "signature songs," the ones that forever after will transport their hearers to a specific time and place. The first, courtesy of Irving Berlin, was the car-trip song, the one my mother and oldest sister sang whenever we left town. My sister at the wheel, my mother in the passenger seat, the two of them swapped roles in a syncopated show tune that required concentration and perfect pitch:

I hear music but there's no one there
I smell blossoms but the trees are bare...

In the backseat, we three littlest girls tapped our feet and asked for that song again and again.

The second one, of uncertain provenance, anchors me not to a place and time, exactly, but to the feeling of my mother's presence. It's an old campfire song that begins:

Tell me why the stars do shine
Tell me why the ivy twines …

My mother liked listening to the radio, and my earliest memories place her in the kitchen, singing along to "Autumn Leaves." We have a recording of her singing "Flow Gently, Sweet Afton," her voice dear and steady and wholly earnest, even with her brother teasing her in the background, groaning theatrically as the seventh stanza commences.

We were musical girls. Why did we not think to sing?

Until eight years ago, Ellen's work focused mainly on children moving from foster care toward adoption; even then, transition was her specialty and music her chief tool. The addition of hospice work arrived through the unlikely conduit of her mother's physical resilience. While making a full recovery from breast cancer, Ruth took Ellen along to a health conference, where the woman at the reception desk, who knew of Ellen's work with children and music, gave her a long, appraising look. "We need music in hospice," she said, and within weeks Ellen was hunting up music for Annie, the lady who loved birds.

The dying, no matter their fear or confusion, no matter the distraction of pain or will-making or the coming and going of strangers, can make clear their musical desires. After the bird lady came client number two, a day-care owner who whispered from her bed: "Ellen. Please. No children's music." Another woman, young and cancer-stricken, lifted both hands and pattered her fingers: "None of this," she instructed, meaning percussion. Then her hands smoothed out, swooping through the air. "This," she said, meaning strings.

Ellen collects people's wishes and releases them like butterflies, either as live music, when she can, or as recorded music, which she prescribes as medicine, taking as inspiration a doctor she once knew who wrote a literal prescription for a Chopin *étude*. "You've got to get the music into them," she says, as if talking about an IV drip. "They know what they need. The woman who didn't want kids' music? She was an oldies girl. She wanted to go out to the oldies, and that's exactly what she did."

A Healing Touch

Ellen says "go out" instead of "die," swapping the language of hospice for the slang of the music hall. *Hey, folks, you've been a great audience! We're gonna go out to a little tune first recorded in …*

Louise goes out to Hank Williams.

Susie goes out to Bach.

Carleen goes out to a polka.

Frank goes out to a tone piece made up on the spot.

You can almost hear applause from the Other Side.

My mother went out to the sound of four daughters moving gingerly through the house. We were quiet, yes; we knew the end was nigh; but because we were living beings we also had to move, to clang plates down from the cupboard, answer the telephone, turn on a hair dryer, shoo a cat from a table top. I suppose we laughed, at least a little—people do, in spite of everything. One of us tiptoed into her bedroom every few minutes, listened for a while to the metronome of her breathing, then tiptoed out. We murmured things to her—the things you murmur (thank you; I love you). We combed her hair and cooled her brow and held her narrow hands. We roamed through the house, drawing curtains open or shut, letting animals in or out, living an evening that would have been unremarkable except for the remarkable fact of her leaving us. We spoke in cadences that rose and fell, rose and fell, like notes along a scale.

When I begin to wonder how the dying hear, Ellen points me to somebody who just might know: her ex-husband, Rupert, who agrees to tell the miraculous story of his round-trip voyage across the River Jordan.

Ellen begins with the part Rupert can't remember: the phone ringing in her house on a bright Tuesday in September. Ellen and Rupert's son had just gone off to college. She picked up the phone. Bring your son back home, Rupert's family told Ellen. *It looks bad.* At the hospital Ellen found her ex-husband in a coma brought on by an infection in the brain, but in the nightmarish days following his transfer to Dana Farber Cancer Institute in Boston, a worse, underlying diagnosis emerged: acute myelogenous leukemia.

Rupert takes over the narrative now, remembering his coma as something like consciousness—a fuzzy, nonverbal awareness in which he admits that "the light was going out." As Rupert hovered between worlds and his family was told that "it could go either way," his visual field narrowed to encompass no more than a hospital room's overbright ceiling light and its single black screw. His aural field shrank, too, similarly overbright and nearly unbearable: the "yack-yack" of a television set that the nurses kept turned on. He managed at last, swimming toward full consciousness, to communicate his wish for silence, or at least for deliverance from a certain kind of noise. After that, his loved ones started bringing in music.

The next sound he recalls with any clarity emanated from a Paul Winter CD called *Earth Mass*, a blend of choral music and sounds from nature, a secular liturgy that found Rupert (he believes now that it was *aimed* at him) through the fog. A piece called "Mystery" moved him especially: "Whatever my head had been thinking about—deities and spirituality—that one piece of music articulated how I felt about a higher power as well as anything ever could." Even now, healthy and healed, his composure falters when he describes how that music connected him with the Great Unknowable at the very moment when he felt most human. "We all have these unique chords that represent our—our interiors," Rupert tells me, his voice filled with a becalmed awe. "Inside each of us there's this rhythm and blues"—here he chuckles at himself—"yes, this rhythm and blues that gets reverberated and released by sound. And it brings you to a place of joy."

Then Rupert addresses side B, giving grief its due. "I never thought of it as listening to my own funeral music," he says, in answer to my question, "but so much of the music I love is filled with sadness." He mentions Barber's "Adagio for Strings" and Celtic music in general, all that sweet lamentation. And bagpipes, oh yeah. "Life is about paradox," he reminds me; certain music "undoes" us because it simultaneously calls up our grief and allows for its release. Rupert believes he got sick in part because of old, unmet losses, and it's hard to argue with a guy who rowed the boat ashore, then back again.

For Ellen, Rupert's long and bumpy journey back to health was like a set of instructions that urged her ever deeper into the hospice work that would come to define so much of her practice. She had shared a life with Rupert once, and she understood what music meant to him.

The dying hear us. Rupert's experience bears that out, and I'm glad for it as I follow Ellen into a charmless room overstuffed with clanking nursing-home furniture. Everything here is crank-upable and crankdownable, producing metallically bright sounds, hard on the ears. This is no sun-buttered bedroom in the family homestead, the kind of setting where one might, in Ellen's words, "die beautifully."

We are here to see Caroline, eighty-seven years old, afflicted by Alzheimer's, erstwhile singer of cowboy songs, long-ago player of guitar. I'd hoped for a tone piece, but Caroline's a bluegrass gal. One week ago, before her sudden decline, Caroline played a harmonica for Ellen and all, intermittently singing "yes yes yes yes"; but today she has gone deeply asleep. Her metronomic breathing tells the tale. Ellen plots a course to the bed, leans down, and murmurs, "Hey, cowboy girl. It's Ellen. I brought you some music." On the other side of the bed, squashed into chairs between the bedrail and the window, sit Caroline's daughters, Rose and Susan, and Susan's husband, Herbert, who's working a crossword puzzle. They raise their pleasant faces, expectant and a little nervous, as if they'd accepted free tickets but forgot to ask the name of the show.

We shed our coats and purses, and as Ellen wrests her guitar from its slipcase, I search out a place to stow our things. The room houses two women, its blueprint cut into miserly sections by ash-pink curtains that jangle open and closed along metal tracks. Caroline's roommate, Hannah, sits on her bed, deaf and wide-eyed, about twelve inches from a loud and glimmering

TV. Behind Hannah's curtain I perceive an alcove, part of a third adjustable table, and a baffling jumble-sale heap of children's toys: dolls and tea sets and pretend diaper bags and baby clothes. Behind that, a shut door that hides a closet or bathroom or maybe another room like this one: humid and claustrophobic, smelling of chicken patties and disinfectant and human deterioration.

As I slide through the space between the foot of Hannah's bed and the side of Caroline's bed, intending to stash our coats on the table behind the curtain, I discover, amazingly, another roommate, a dumpling of a woman sitting next to her bed, bent at the waist and flopped over like a folded pillow. Her dark hair flows groundward. She is either asleep, or meditating, or intently studying her large, spatulate, unshod feet. It crosses my mind that she might even be dead, but that's more than I can wrestle with presently, too felled by the tableau I've walked into: a dying woman attended by daughters. My mission, reassembled as urgently as Chuck's shelving units, is simply to get through.

From the television commences a chirruping version of "Auld Lang Syne" performed by a quintet of muppets. Ellen, who'll use whatever's handy, finds the key on her guitar and joins in. It's kind of cheerful, actually, cute and hummable, and so I hum along help-lessly, looking around. A pink flyswatter decorates one wall, and on another hangs a bulletin board with a single item pinned to its lower quarter: a five-inch-square greeting card broadcasting a single, filigreed word: JOY.

After the muppets conclude their New Year's bene-diction, Ellen murmurs a few more words to Caroline, who, I now believe, hears all. A nurse comes in to bring us snacks and turn down the television. Susan delivers her homework, a long list of songs her mother once loved, heavy on gospel and the kind of plunk-a-plunk standards beloved by self-taught guitar players of a certain era. Ellen begins, more or less on her own, with "Home on the Range." But really, there is something about music, even in a place such as this—maybe especially in a place such as this—that's irresistible. The next song down is "I'll Fly Away," one of Caroline's favorites, and one of mine, too. Ellen strums softly, taking the melody. I add the high harmony—what else can I do?—and there it is, that "inner chord" Rupert spoke of, the place that houses grief and joy. With two voices, the song takes on layers and motion as Susan, pulled by the tide of sound, adds the low harmony, so now we are three, and by song's end both daughters are in, and here's the surprise: they're wonderful. Susan sings in a sweet, steady vibrato, and Rose turns in one of those between-the-harmony lines that church-trained singers do so well. "Wow," I marvel, "where did that come from?" And the women tell of performances, forty years past, a trio with their mother—church music, big surprise—in three-part harmony. There's another sister—she'll arrive later in the day—who sang, too. We ask them to do a little number, but they demur, claiming themselves dusty with disuse. Ellen, perhaps sensing an irreplaceable chance, launches into "Amazing Grace," and by the end of the first measure the song has lured us all, including Herbert, who puts down his puzzle and sings gorgeously, eyes closed. Our blended notes rise up and up and widen the room and the world, yes they do. Ellen has barely taken her eyes from Caroline this whole time, and her focus finally pulls me there, to the frail, opalescent face that takes in the music, you can see it, amazing indeed: a gradual softening, like a shade being drawn gently down against a too-bright day.

Everybody sees this, and now we're a team, lighting into the rest of the songs, including one about blackflies penned by Caroline herself as a young wife, a ditty sung to the tune of "Roll Out the Barrel." "Roll out the fly dope," we sing, Rose and Susan reading the lyrics off a wrinkled sheet, "'cause the swarm's all heeeeere!"

After my mother died—that very evening—one of my sisters opened a can of yellow paint. The mattress had disappeared from the bed; I don't know how or when, though I think I remember us muscling the new one through the door. How the paint materialized is another mystery: it was Sunday night in a small town and nothing was open. Maybe I've gotten the day wrong, and I mean the evening of her wake, or her funeral; days around a death tend to mingle kaleidoscopically. I watched my sister open the paint with a screwdriver, pour it into a pan, and attack the bedroom walls with a roller. Finally, the rest of us helped, rollers all around, implying, with every wild stroke: Nobody died here. After the paint dried, the shade recalled the color of our mother's skin at the last.

At Caroline's bedside, we sing for a very long time. Spirituals and dirges and cowboy songs, a lullaby, some Christmas carols, a few old-fashioned hymns. Caroline breathes and breathes, her fragile features peaceful and unchanging. I've begun to think of this as praying, as holy work. We are a ring of people, an ad hoc band of angels—*blue angels, blue angels*—mingling our voices, magnificently I believe, except for an odd, intermittent, discordant note. First I hear it, then I think I've imagined it, then it pops up again, there, like the lowing of a cow. At first I suspect Herbert, but he's right here, eyes closed, in key, smoothing into "Swing Low, Sweet Chariot" as if he's sung it all his life—which, as it turns out, he has. I glance around for a blinky intercom, or a radiator on the fritz, trying to pin the sound to something inanimate. We sing "Down by the Riverside," then "Michael Row the Boat Ashore," and there it is again, that note—thudding and unharmonious, and it's coming from behind me, from behind the pink curtain, where the little dumpling woman—whom I have completely forgotten; who has a name; whose name is Maggie—is still sitting, still folded in half, singing.

I catch Susan's eye and point toward the curtain. "Maggie," Susan calls, "is that you?"

Comes the voice, the same lowing: "Can't help it. I know 'em all."

We all laugh, something new gets released, and our choir increases by one. When a nurse arrives to wheel Maggie off to lunch, I realize that head-over-knees is the permanent shape of her body. Hannah gets wheeled out next, and now it's just us, munching crackers, chatting amiably. The music has made us friends. Susan and Rose tell tales on their mother, who was a hoot, a real ticket, her life one big fat yes. They recall the house up north, all that churchgoing and fly-swatting and outhouse visiting and snow shoveling. This, too, this rise and fall of sisters talking—this, too, thank God, sounds like music. Their mother sleeps.

Early the next day, Ellen calls to tell me she returned to Caroline's room a few hours later with a CD of bluegrass gospel, many of the songs an encore of the morning's bedside chorus. Caroline went out to the sound of Alison Krauss, dying before day's end.

"Do you think her daughters—" I hesitate, hoping I know the answer. "Do you think her daughters would have sung without us?"

"What do you think?"

"I think they wouldn't have."

A day later—mothers and daughters still in my head—I call Ellen back to ask a question that's been burbling beneath the surface since our October chat on her mother's sun-whitened beach.

"Have you thought about what you'd provide for Ruth? If her time comes in the way Caroline's did?"

Missing my meaning, Ellen considers possibilities for funeral music.

"I don't mean after," I explain. "I mean during. If she, you know, if she lingers."

After a long pause, Ellen decides, "My mother won't be a lingerer. I just don't see her going out that way."

We didn't see our mother going out that way, either. Nor did Susan and Rose see it for the woman who sang about blackflies at the top of her lungs. I try again, because I really want to know. "But if she does? Linger, I mean?"

Uncharacteristically, Ellen has trouble meeting me here, in this conversation that rests on the unthinkable. Ellen, whose every day is filled with musical goodbyes, cannot countenance her own mother's final parting.

Which is a stupendous relief to me, a tidal release. We did not sing to our mother—we musical girls—not because we didn't think to, but because we couldn't bear to.

But music is contagious; people who love to sing will sing. Strike the harp, they'll join the chorus every time. Maggie sang from her folded body with a view of her own feet. Rose and Susan sang into their sadness; Herbert put aside his puzzle to pray inside a song.

A Healing Touch

If someone like Ellen had asked, my sisters and I would have produced a long list: the car-trip song, the campfire song, "Autumn Leaves," "Flow Gently Sweet Afton" and more, so many more. "Pardon Me Boys" and "Danny Boy" and "The Boy Who Wore the Blue." "Rock of Ages" and "I Am a Rock" and "Rock Around the Clock." Folk songs, show tunes, Latin hymns, Elvis. If someone like Ellen had started us off, we could have kept it up for days.

If Ellen ever finds herself voiceless at a bedside—if that unimaginable evening comes to pass—I hope a blue angel, blue angel flies into the room. Someone kind and fearless and made of music. Someone who can signal those first, painful, quavering notes, familiar and irresistible, to help a grieving daughter tell her sorrow in a song.

ABOUT THE CONTRIBUTORS

GERRY BOYLE was born in Chicago, raised in Rhode Island, and now lives in China, Maine. He has worked as a journalist and columnist for Maine newspapers, but is most known for his Jack McMorrow crime novels, which include *Deadline, Potshot, Pretty Dead,* and *Home Body.*

WESLEY MCNAIR has published volumes of poems, essays, and three anthologies of Maine writing. He has received grants from the Fulbright and Guggenheim foundations, two NEA and two Rockefeller Fellowships, and a United States Artist Ford Fellowship. He lives with his wife Diane in Mercer, Maine.

BILL ROORBACH, a resident of Farmington, Maine, has received an NEA fellowship, an O. Henry Award, and the Flannery O'Connor Award for his collection of stories, *Big Bend.* He has published a novel, *The Smallest Color,* and three volumes of nonfiction, most recently *Temple Stream.* His work has appeared in *The Atlantic, Harper's,* and many other periodicals.

RICHARD RUSSO, of Camden, Maine, has produced several volumes of fiction, among them *The Risk Pool,*

Straight Man, Nobody's Fool, and *Empire Falls,* for which he won the Pulitzer Prize. He has also written for the movies and television. His latest novel is *Bridge of Sighs.*

SUSAN STERLING is a volunteer with Hospice Volunteers of the Waterville Area. Her essays and stories have appeared in *The New York Times, The Christian Science Monitor,* and various literary journals, and have been anthologized in *The Best American Sports Writing 1998, The Berkeley Women's Literary Revolution,* and *The Way Life Should Be: Stories by Contemporary Maine Writers.* She lives with her husband, Paul Machlin, in Waterville, Maine.

MONICA WOOD, from Portland, Maine, has published her stories in numerous magazines and anthologies; moreover, they have been presented on Public Radio International and awarded the Pushcart Prize. She has published three novels, including *Any Bitter Thing;* a book of linked stories, *Ernie's Ark;* and two volumes for writers, most recently *The Pocket Muse.*